Ace the CMC®!

You Can Do It!

Cardiac Medicine Certification Study Guide

Nicole Kupchik
MN, RN, CCNS, CCRN-CMC, PCCN-K

Nicole Kupchik Consulting, Inc.
Seattle, WA

Copyright © 2023 Nicole Kupchik

Ace the CMC®: You Can Do It!
Cardiac Medicine Certification Study Guide

All rights reserved. No part of this publication may be reproduced, distributed, or transmitted in any form or by any means, including photocopying, recording, or other electronic or mechanical methods, without the prior written permission of the publisher, except in the case of brief quotations embodied in critical reviews and certain other noncommercial uses permitted by copyright law. For permission requests, write to the publisher, addressed "Attention: Permissions Coordinator," at the address below.

ISBN: 978-0-9978349-9-4

This book is protected under the seal of the United States Copyright Office in accordance with title 17, Registration Number TX 8-652-353.

Front cover image by O'Daniel Designs.
Book design by Gorham Printing, Inc.

First printing edition 2018.

Nicole Kupchik
P.O. Box 15900
Seattle, WA 98115

www.nicolekupchikconsulting.com

Special thanks...

My mom, Carol who passed away in 2019

My many amazing friends—
you all know who you are!

Helen Wing—I wouldn't have survived
the past 7 years without you!

Gina O'Daniel

Dr. Elizabeth Bridges—
My continual mentor

Ashley—my co-conspirator in discussing everything
business and female empowerment. You inspire me.

My pals at Harborview, Swedish & Overlake
who have always encouraged me over the years!

And the THOUSANDS of nurses who have attended my classes,
given constructive feedback & took the exams.
You are all an inspiration to me!

The encouragement you all have given me
is immeasurable and completely appreciated!

Unless we are making
progress in our nursing
every year, every month, every week,
take my word for it,
we are going back.

—Florence Nightingale (May 1872)

Contents

A note of encouragement from Nicole vii

Thank you to the contributors viii

About the CMC® Subspecialty Exam xi

The CMC® Test Plan xii

Chapter 1 Cardiac Basics 1

Chapter 2 Acute Coronary Syndrome
with Medication Table 7

Chapter 3 Hemodynamic Monitoring 35

Chapter 4 Heart Failure & Cardiomyopathies 55

Chapter 5 Valvular Dysfunction, Inflammatory Diseases
& Other Cardiac Issues 71

Chapter 6 Arrhythmias & Cardiac Arrest 85

Chapter 7 Vascular Issues 107

Chapter 8 Other Patient Care Problems 115

CMC Quizzes with Answers & Rationale 155

References 231

About the author 233

You Can Do It!

A note of encouragement from Nicole

Congratulations on taking steps to becoming certified and obtaining the CMC® subspecialty certification!

In 2002, I passed the CCRN® for the first time. I am going to let you in on a little secret. I was eligible to sit the exam in 1994. I attended three certification review courses before taking the exam. Why? I lacked confidence and was so afraid of failing. I finally got up the courage in 2002 and aced it!

I can distinctly remember walking out of the testing site questioning myself and why I waited so long to take it. I had so much self-doubt. It was a little crazy, because clinically, I was confident. A couple years later I started teaching sections of the exam at Harborview and in 2006 started co-teaching the prep courses nationally.

Who would think someone could go from having a complete lack of confidence to teaching the courses a few years later? Mental mindset is everything. I want you to tell yourself every day that you can do this!!!

I often hear nurses say "becoming certified doesn't make you a better nurse." I completely disagree with statements like that. The journey you will take in preparing to become certified increases your knowledge to better care for your patients. I truly believe every nurse should be certified in their specialty.

The CMC® exam was my next professional goal & certification to achieve. Again, I was so scared to take the exam, but did and passed with flying colors. Being prepared is the key to becoming certified. I was so proud to obtain this subspecialty certification.

I was inspired to publish this book by nurses who attended my review courses. Many of the study books available are overwhelming & contain too much information. My goal is always to break down disease states into digestible pieces so you can learn & understand the content. I did this for the CCRN® & PCCN® and I wanted to offer a review book for the CMC®.

My biggest piece of advice to you in studying is, of course to understand different conditions, but do as many practice test questions as possible. Read the rationales for questions you get right & those you miss. I believe that is the key to success. You can do it!

Thank you to the following contributors:

Michelle A. Dedeo DNP, ARNP-CNS, ACCNS-AG, CCRN, CNRN, SCRN

Michelle received her Bachelors of Science in Nursing from the University of Wisconsin Madison and her Masters in Nursing and Doctorate in Nursing Practice from the University of Washington. She is the Neuroscience Clinical Nurse Specialist at Providence Swedish in Seattle, WA.

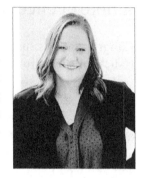

James "Charlie" Edwards MSN-ED, RN, NPD-BC, CCRN-K, CEN

Charlie earned a Bachelor of Science in Nursing from the University of Phoenix and a Master of Science in Nursing Education from Western Governors University. He has been a nurse for over 30 years and is currently the Director of Nursing Professional Development at Desert Regional Medical Center in Palm Springs, California.

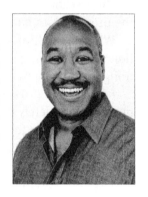

Kelly King DNP, MN, RN, CCRN

Kelly received her Bachelors of Science in Nursing from Bradley University, a Masters in Nursing from the University of Washington and a Doctorate of Nursing Practice from Rush University. She currently works as a critical care nurse at Rush University Medical Center.

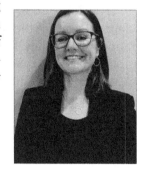

Kristin Nathan MNE, RN, CCRN-K

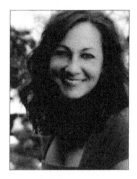

Kristin Nathan has been a registered nurse, specializing in critical care, post open heart recovery and resuscitation, for 25 years. She graduated with her BSN in 1995 from The Ohio State University and completed her Masters in Nursing Education from Oregon Health & Sciences University in 2019. She currently works as a Nursing Education and Simulation Specialist for Legacy Health Medical Center in Portland, Oregon.

Kristin has worked as a clinical adjunct faculty at Linfield Good Samaritan School of Nursing and has been a clinical unit educator for many years in a cardiovascular ICU. She has developed an open-heart training program and protocols related to care management with post open heart recovery and is certified in cardiac surgery advanced life support. Kristin has spoken nationally on advanced hemodynamics and promoting CCRN certification. Kristin also collaborates with the Greater Portland Chapter of AACN speaking on hemodynamics for their statewide critical care nursing consortium and is a co-facilitator for Legacy Health critical care orientation program.

Dr. Todd D. Ray DNP, ARNP, ACNP-BC, RN

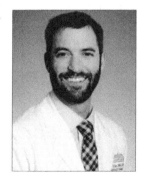

Todd received his Bachelors of Science in Zoology from the University of Idaho, and his Bachelors of Science in Nursing from Lewis-Clark State College. He completed his Masters in Nursing and Doctorate in Nursing Practice from the University of Washington. He currently works at Harborview Medical Center for the Division of Pulmonary Critical Care and Sleep Medicine, co-directs the Medical ICU Quality Improvement Program, and teaches at Seattle University as an Adjunct Professor for the Acute care doctoral nurse practitioner program.

Amy Stafford MN, APRN, CCNS

Amy received her Bachelors of Science in Nursing from Saint Joseph's College of Maine and her Masters in Nursing from the University of Washington School of Nursing. She has over 25 years of experience working in critical care in various capacities. She is currently the Clinical Nurse Specialist for critical care at Maine Medical Center in Portland, ME.

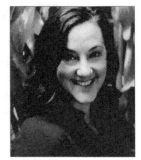

Joel Green MSN, RN, CCRN-CMC-CSC

Joel Green lives in Seattle, Washington. He received his BS in Nursing from Northwest University. He later received his MSN in Healthcare Education from University of Phoenix and was inducted into Sigma Theta Tau. Joel has also completed some post masters doctoral work through Vanderbilt University. Currently, Joel is working an Assistant Nurse Manager in a Cardiothoracic surgical ICU in Seattle. He has worked in telemetry, cardio thoracic ICU, medical ICU, and post anesthesia care units. He has also worked for several medical device companies as an educator.

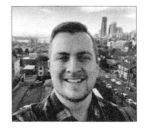

About the CMC® Subspecialty Exam

The CMC® is administered by the American Association of Critical Care Nurses (AACN). Their website information is: www.aacn.org

Qualifications to sit the exam:

- Hold a current unencumbered nursing license
- A current nursing certification to which the CMC will be attached.
  - Must be nationally accredited
  - Example: CCRN, PCCN, CCNS
- Practice as a RN or APRN for 1,750 hours in direct care of adult patients; 875 care of acutely/critically ill adult cardiac medicine **OR**
- RN or APRN with 5 years experience, minimum of 2,000 hours, 144 in most recent year.
- If you have any questions about eligibility, please contact AACN—they are super helpful!

The application includes demographic information and an honor statement. You will need to provide the name & contact information of a colleague who can verify your eligibility.

Once AACN receives your application, they usually take about 1-2 weeks to process it. Once it has been processed & you are deemed eligible, you will receive an email from AACN with directions to schedule your exam. You have 180 days to sit the exam. Easy peasy!

The CMC® exam consists of 90 questions. Fifteen questions will not count toward your final score. They are used for statistical data for future exams. It's kind of a bummer you don't know which questions don't count. The advice I ALWAYS give nurses—if you come across a question that you have NO idea the answer, tell yourself it's a question that doesn't count. Don't psych yourself out if you don't know the answer. There will be some questions that you won't be completely sure.

Exam questions are written at the application & analysis levels based on the Synergy model of care; meaning they aren't super basic questions. They want to assess your knowledge in taking care of patients & what to anticipate in treatment. On that same thought, they also aren't trying to trick you. Each question will have 4 answer choices & only one is the correct answer.

You will have 2 hours to complete the exam. The passing "cut score" is 50 out of 75. Translated—you have to get about 67% correct to pass. You can easily do this but, you need to prepare & study. The way they score is a little more complicated than a straight 67%, but I'm not completely sure exactly how that's done.

AACN Test Plan—CMC®

Cardiovascular Conditions (23%)
Non-Cardiovascular Conditions (23%)
Therapeutic interventions (39%)
Monitoring & Diagnostics (16%)

Cardiovascular Conditions (23%)

Cardiac Conditions
- Acute coronary syndrome
  - (e.g., STEMI, NSTEMI, unstable angina)
- Cardiac tamponade
- Cardiomyopathies
- Dysrhythmias
- Heart failure
- Hypertensive urgency or emergency
- Inflammatory and infectious conditions
- Pericardial effusion
- Pulmonary edema
- Syncope
- Valvular disorders

Vascular Conditions
- Acute arterial occlusion
- Acute venous thrombosis
- Aortic aneurysm or dissection
- Hyperlipidemia
- Post-intervention vascular complication

Non-Cardiovascular Conditions (23%)

Respiratory
- Acute pulmonary embolus
- Acute respiratory failure (e.g., ARDS, ALI)
- Pleural space abnormalities (e.g., pneumothorax)
- Pulmonary hypertension
- Sleep apnea

Endocrine
- Adrenal disorders
- Diabetes mellitus
- Metabolic syndrome
- Thyroid disorders

Hematology
- Coagulopathies
- Anemia

Neurology
- Cerebrovascular accident (stroke)

Renal
- Acute kidney injury
- Chronic kidney disease
- Electrolyte imbalances

Multisystem
- Multisystem organ dysfunction syndrome (MODS)
- Shock states
- Non-cardiac chest pain

Therapeutic Interventions (39%)

Cardiac Procedures
- Right heart catheterization
- Left heart catheterization
- Percutaneous coronary interventions
- Pericardiocentesis
- Intra-aortic balloon pumps
- Left ventricular assist devices (LVADs)
- Percutaneous structural heart interventions

Vascular Interventions
- Peripheral angiography and interventions
- Carotid angiography and interventions
- Endovascular grafts
- Catheter-directed thrombolysis

Cardiovascular Pharmacology
- Anti-dysrhythmics
- Anticoagulants
- Diuretics
- Inotropes
- Platelet inhibitors
- Thrombolytics
- Vasoactive agents

Respiratory
- Non-invasive ventilation
- Mechanical ventilation

Electrophysiologic Interventions
- Temporary pacemakers
- Permanent pacemakers
- Cardiac resynchronization therapy
- Implantable cardioverter defibrillator
- External wearable defibrillator
- Ablation
- Cardioversion
- Defibrillation

Renal
- Renal replacement therapy
  - (e.g., hemodialysis, CRRT, SCUF)

Multisystem
- Targeted temperature management
- Palliative and end-of-life care

Monitoring & Diagnostics (16%)

Cardiovascular
- Hemodynamic monitoring
- Echocardiography
- Electrocardiography (ECG)
- Laboratory testing
- Stress testing
- Remote cardiovascular monitoring
  - » (e.g., dysrhythmia monitoring, pulmonary artery sensor)

Respiratory
- Arterial blood gases (ABG)
- Mixed venous gases
- Pulse oximetry
- End-tidal capnography (EtCO2)
- Radiography

GENERAL TEST TIPS:

✓ Go in with a confident attitude! You can do this!

✓ Get to the testing site 30 min before your test time

✓ Answer every question

✓ You can change answers, but…**DON'T**!!

✓ You'll have a clock on the bottom of your computer screen, pace yourself

✓ Read the question and try to guess the answer before looking at the options

✓ You will find out right away if you passed!

Mental Attitude is **Everything**!

You Can Do It!

Chapter 1

Cardiac Basics

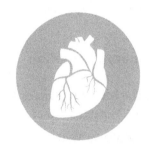

Cardiac Basics

Coronary Artery Perfusion

- » Both the right & left **coronary arteries** arise at the base of the aorta (Sinus of Valsalva); immediately above the aortic valve

- » Two main coronary arteries: right & left

- » Coronary arteries are perfused during…?
  - DIASTOLE!
  - This is why tachycardia is so challenging in heart failure & ACS
  - Tachycardia decreases perfusion time & diastolic filling time

Coronary Circulation

- » The **RIGHT Coronary Artery (RCA)** perfuses the:
  - *Inferior Wall
  - Right atrium
  - Right ventricle
  - Posterior wall in ~ 90% of the population
  - Back of the septum
  - SA Node
  - AV Node

- » The **LEFT Main Artery** perfuses the left side of the heart
  - Think *MAJOR PUMP!*
  - Nickname (if vessel is occluded) = WIDOW MAKER!!!

The **Left Main Artery** bifurcates into the:

- » Left Anterior Descending (LAD) Artery &

- » Left Circumflex Artery

Cardiac Basics

The LAD perfuses the:

- *Septal & Anterior Wall
- Front & bottom of left ventricle
- Front of septum
- Most of the right & left bundles
- Anterior papillary muscle of the mitral valve
- Distal bundle of his

The Left Circumflex perfuses the:

- *Lateral Wall
- Left atrium
- Back of left ventricle
- Posterior wall in ~ 10% to 15% of the population

Atrial contraction

- Contributes about 20 – 25% of cardiac output
- SO, when patients go into atrial fibrillation, they lose that **atrial kick!**
- In low EF states/heart failure, they may not tolerate loss of atrial kick so well!

Preload

The initial stretching of the myocardium prior to contraction; therefore, it is related to the sarcomere length at the end of diastole.

- Equated to volume status (with caution!)
- High preload = Fluid overload (But not always clinically true!)
- Low preload = Fluid deficit (Again, not always true!)
- Pulmonary Artery Catheter measures preload on the:
  - Right side of the heart as the central venous pressure "CVP" or right atrial pressure "RAP"
  - Left side of the heart as the pulmonary artery occlusive pressure or "PAOP"

Afterload

» The **resistance** the ventricles have to overcome to eject blood

» High afterload = **Vasoconstriction**

» Low afterload = **Vasodilation**

Heart Sounds

Valvular Auscultation Points:

» Aortic valve: Right sternal border, 2nd ICS

» Pulmonic valve: Left sternal border, 2nd ICS

» Tricuspid valve: Left sternal border, 4 - 5th ICS

» Mitral valve: left mid-clavicular line, 5th ICS

Normal Heart Sounds

» S_1: closure of the mitral & tricuspid valves
- Systole
- Loudest over mitral area
- 1/3 of the cardiac cycle

» S_2: closure of pulmonic & aortic valve
- Diastole
- Loudest over aortic area, 2nd ICS
- 2/3 of the cardiac cycle

Extra Heart Sounds

» S_3: Ventricular Gallop
- Auscultated in fluid overload; when preload is elevated
- Normal in kids, high cardiac output, 3rd trimester of pregnancy
- Listen over apex area
- "Ken-tuck-y" or "I Believe" cadence

- » S_4: Atrial gallop (pre-systolic)
  - Sound caused by vibration of atria ejecting into non-compliant ventricles
  - Auscultated during ischemia (increased resistance to ventricular filling)
  - Other causes: Ischemia, HTN, pulmonary stenosis, CAD, Aortic stenosis, left ventricular hypertrophy
  - Listen over tricuspid or mitral area
  - "Ten-ne-see" or "Believe-me" cadence
- » **Split Heart Sounds**
  - When one valve closes later than the other
    - ▷ **Best heard during <u>inspiration</u>
  - Split S_1 - Mitral closes before tricuspid valve
    - ▷ RBBB or PVCs or ventricular pacing (think wide QRS, ventricular dyssynchrony)
  - Split S_2 - Aortic closes before pulmonic valve
    - ▷ Overfilled right ventricle
    - ▷ Atrial septal defect (ASD)

Heart Valves

AV Valves:

» Mitral (on the left) & tricuspid (on the right) & are:

» Closed during - SYSTOLE!

» Open during - DIASTOLE!

Semilunar Valves

» Aortic (on the left) & pulmonic (on the right) & are:

» Open during - SYSTOLE!

» Closed during - DIASTOLE!

You Can Do It!

Chapter 2

Acute Coronary Syndrome

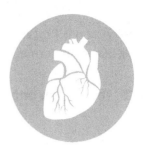

Topics covered in this chapter include:

- ACS risk factors
- Angina
- Non-ST segment elevation myocardial infarction (NSTEMI or NSTE-ACS)
- ST segment elevation myocardial infarction (STEMI or STE-ACS)
- Medications used in ACS
- 12 Lead ECG
- Types of MIs
- Conduction defects & heart block
- Complications of MI (pericarditis, papillary muscle rupture, ventricular septal rupture)
- Cardiogenic shock
- Cardiogenic pulmonary edema
- Cardiac medication reference table

Acute Coronary Syndrome (ACS)

Pathophysiology: Progressive atherosclerosis with or without plaque rupture causing blood clot formation leading to an imbalance of O_2 supply & demand

In ACS, there is an imbalance of oxygen supply & demand

O_2 Supply:

- Coronary arteries
- Diastolic filling time
- Cardiac output
- Hemoglobin
- SaO_2/ SpO_2

O_2 Demand:

- Heart rate
- Contractility
- Preload
- Afterload

Cardiac Risk Factors

Non-modifiable:

- Age
- Gender
- Family history
- Race

Modifiable:

- Smoking
- Hyperlipidemia
- Obesity
- Diabetes mellitus
- Diet
- Physical inactivity
- Hypertension

Cardiac Biomarkers:

- » Troponin-I (or T) most sensitive & specific
  - New AHA recommendations to only do Troponin-I
  - Isoenzymes are a waste of $$$
- » Elevates in 3 - 6 hours
- » Peaks in 14 - 20 hours
- » Returns to normal in 1 - 2 weeks

- » Most labs > 0.4 ng/mL is considered elevated
- » Usually do 3 Troponin-I levels every 8 hours OR check until you see a peak & decline, then stop checking them!
- » Many facilities are using high-sensitivity troponin (hs-cTn)

ACS Symptoms:

Chest pain/symptom assessment—ask these questions (OLDCART)

- » **O**nset?
- » **L**ocation?
- » **D**uration?
- » **C**haracteristics?
- » **A**ssociated s/s?
- » **R**elieving factors?
- » **T**reatment?

Remember not everyone presents the same way!

- » Caucasian males may present with midsternal chest pain radiating to the left arm & jaw
- » Females commonly present with GI symptoms, back pain or fatigue
- » Diabetics have neuropathies & may not feel pain!
  - They often present with shortness of breath

Non-cardiac chest pain causes:

- » Pleuritic pain – worse with inspiration & exhalation
  - Pulmonary embolism & pleurisy
- » Gastrointestinal discomfort – GERD
- » Gastroenteritis
- » Stomach ulcers
- » Gallbladder
- » Esophageal spasms
- » Pancreatitis

NSTE-ACS (Angina)

- » Stable
  - Exertional; symptoms cease when exertion stops
  - May have a fixed vessel stenosis with demand ischemia
  - May require sublingual NTG
- » Unstable
  - Increasing frequency, intensity, time & duration
  - Sign & precursor to a MI
  - 10 - 20% have a myocardial infarction
  - May develop while at rest
  - May require intervention to relieve symptoms
  - Consider antiplatelet therapy (i.e. aspirin)
  - Troponin does not elevate
- » Variant (Prinzmetal's)
  - Sudden pain caused from **coronary artery vasospasm**
  - Occurs at rest or when sleeping
  - Treat with NTG & Calcium Channel Blockers to relieve spasm
    - ▷ Isosorbide dinitrate or mononitrate & Diltiazem
  - **Get 12 Lead ECG with & without symptoms!
  - Will see ST segment changes with pain & symptoms

NSTE-ACS (NSTEMI)

- » <u>Partial occlusion</u> of coronary artery

- » Pain or symptoms may occur at rest & last > 20 min
  - **Hallmark sign pain/symptoms with ↑ frequency, heaviness or pressure

- » Cardiac biomarkers elevated (Troponin-I)

- » 12 lead ECG: ST depression or T wave inversion

- » ST depression or T wave inversion = ischemia
  - ECG changes in different leads in NSTE-ACS are not artery specific like STEMI
  - 8 or more leads with ST depression/T wave inversion & ST elevation in lead aVR, high suspicion for:
    ▷ Proximal LAD occlusion
    ▷ Left main occlusion
    ▷ Multi-vessel disease

- » Treatment: PCI; Early PCI if high risk

ST Elevation MI (STEMI)

- » Emergency!

- » <u>Complete occlusion</u>

- » Treatment: Immediate reperfusion
  - Door to balloon time = < 90 min
  - Cath lab for PCI (preferred) or
  - If Cath lab is not readily available – fibrinolytics, then Cath lab when appropriate

- » Cause: Plaque rupture leading to blood clot formation
  - Platelets aggregate to the atherosclerotic site
  - Occlusive thrombus formation
  - + Cardiac biomarkers (Troponin-I)

  **Hallmark signs—Chest pain/symptoms > 20 min, SOB, diaphoresis

ST Elevation = Injury

- » ≥ 1 mm (limb leads) or ≥ 2 mm (precordial leads)
- » In 2 or more contiguous leads
  - Leads that look at the same wall of the heart
- » New left BBB in precordial leads – suspicious for MI

Timing of ECG Changes

- » **Immediate:** T wave elevates, ST ↑ in leads over the area of infarction
- » **Several hours:** After revascularization, ST normalizes, T waves invert
- » **Several hours – days:** Q waves may develop, reduced R waves, low voltage R wave (sometimes for life)

Emergent MI Medication Treatment:

Aspirin

- » 81 mg – 325 mg PO load – CHEWED!
  - Rectal may be used if unable to take PO
  - DO NOT use enteric coated aspirin
- » Onset of action 1 – 7.5 minutes when chewed
- » Inhibits cyclooxygenase-1 within platelets & prevents formation of thromboxane A_2
- » Disables platelet aggregation
- » Monitor for intolerance & bleeding
- » Used indefinitely post MI
- » Maintenance dose at least 81 mg daily
- » No other NSAIDs for 6 weeks post MI
  - Increases risk of myocardial rupture

Nitroglycerin (NTG)

» 0.4 mg SL every 5 minutes x 3

» Sublingual or spray then initiate infusion (Tridil) if ongoing symptoms

» May use IV if continued chest discomfort/symptoms

» Potent vasodilator

» Monitor for hypotension & headache

» **Reduces preload** & ventricular wall tension

» Decreases myocardial O_2 consumption

» Caution with inferior wall MI
  - Due to hypotension & preload reduction
  - Avoid if suspected right ventricular infarction

» Always ask if they have taken Viagra or Cialis
  - Can lead to significant vasodilation & hypotension!

Oxygen

» **Supplemental O_2 only if SpO_2 < 90%**

» Hyperoxemia can perpetuate oxidative injury after MI
  - There is some evidence it may actually worsen infarct size

» Not needed for patients without evidence of respiratory distress (AHA guideline)

Morphine

» Small incremental doses (1 – 2 mg) IV Q 5 - 15 min if symptoms unrelieved by NTG

» Use as adjunct therapy to NTG

» Potent analgesic & anxiolytic

» Causes venodilation & **reduces preload**

» Decreases workload of heart by also **reducing afterload**

» Use cautiously in UA & NSTEMI!!
  - Increased mortality in a large registry
  - Causes hypotension

» Avoid in right ventricular MI due to preload reduction

Post-PCI Medication Management:

Dual Anti-Platelet Therapy (DAPT)

» For at least 1 year post PCI with stent placement

Aspirin (indefinitely) plus

Thienopyridines (P2 Y_{12} Inhibitors) – with drug eluting stents (DES) or bare metal stents (BMS):

» Plavix (Clopidogrel) 600 mg load; continue 75 mg daily for 12 months <u>or</u>

» Effient (Prasugrel) 60 mg load; continue 10 mg for 12 months <u>or</u>

» Ticagreolor (Brilinta) 180 mg load; 90 mg BID for 12 months
- FYI – Many Cardiologists will load with a $P2Y_{12}$ Inhibitor prior to cath
- Drug duration shorter with BMS

On a case by case analysis, during the PCI the Cardiologist may prescribe:

» Unfractionated Heparin (UFH) <u>or</u>

» Bivalirudin (Angiomax) – during PCI; finish in Cath lab or on unit
- Half-life is 25 min with normal renal function
- Dose: 0.75 mg/kg IV bolus
- Then 1.75 mg/kg/hour IV infusion for duration of the procedure
- May continue for 4 hours post procedure

» GP IIb/IIIa Inhibitors (at time of PCI)
- Abciximab (Reopro)
- Eptifibatide (Integrilin)
- Tirofiban (Aggrastat)
  ▷ Monitor platelet count closely
  ▷ Monitor for bleeding
- **These agents are potent anti-platelet medications!

Post MI with PCI, patients are prescribed "The Big 5"

1) Aspirin (indefinitely)
2) $P2Y_{12}$ Inhibitor (usually for 1 year)
3) Beta blocker (indefinitely)
4) Statin (high dose indefinitely)
5) ACE Inhibitor, ARB or ARNI if EF < 40% (indefinitely)
   - May add Spironolactone, SGLT-2 inhibitor

Beta Blockers: "-olols"

- » Administered within 24 hours if hemodynamically stable, continued indefinitely

- » Hold if hypotension or signs of hypoperfusion/shock

- » Blocks catecholamine & blunts the sympathetic nervous system (SNS)

- » ↓ HR & contractility

- » ↓ myocardial O$_2$ consumption

- » Cardio-protective, ↓ arrhythmias

- » Short and long term, decreases morbidity & mortality

- » Warn patients they may feel exhausted & tired for a few months!
  - Warn of depression
  - Due to SNS blunting
  - Sexual dysfunction

- » Metoprolol (tartrate) & carvedilol mostly used
  - Metoprolol tartrate is the only form of metoprolol that is cardio-protective!

Reminder: Hold the beta blockers in acute exacerbated heart failure!

Statins (HMG CoA Reductase Inhibitors)

- » ↓ cholesterol levels by interfering with body's ability to produce cholesterol by the liver

- » ↓ inflammatory response that theoretically may be responsible for atherosclerotic process

- » Cardio-protective

- » Reduces risk of recurrent MI & stroke

- » Target LDL < 70

- » High dose statins recommended for all patients post MI
  - Examples: Atorvastatin (Lipitor), Rosuvastatin (Crestor), Lovastatin (Mevacor) or Simvastatin (Zocor)
  - Monitor for muscle weakness, myopathies & myositis
  - May accelerate the development of Type 2 diabetes
  - Baseline LFTs
  - Rhabdomyolysis—extremely rare

ACE Inhibitors ("prils") or Angiotensin Receptor Blockers ("sartans")

» EF ≤ 40%, new heart failure

» ↓ intra-cardiac pressures

» Slows cardiac remodeling

» ↓ preload & afterload

» **Commonly prescribed ACE Inhibitors:**
- Lisinopril (Zestril, Prinivil)
- Enalapril (Vasotec)
- Captopril (Capoten)
- Ramipril (Altace)

» **Commonly prescribed ARBs:**
- Valsartan (Diovan)
- Losartan (Cozaar)
- Candesartan (Atacand)
- Olmesartan (Benicar)

Side Effects of ACE Inhibitors & ARBs:

» **Cough – 19%!**
- ACE Inhibitors prevent the breakdown of bradykinin & substance P in the lungs
- Accumulation of protussive mediators
- Use ARB or ARNI instead

» **Hypotension**
- 1st dose effect
- Syncope & dizziness

» **Hyperkalemia**
- Blocking action of aldosterone

» **Renal dysfunction**
- Monitor BUN & creatinine

» **Rash**

» **Angioedema**
- Rare, 0.1 – 0.2% incidence
- Higher incidence in female & African American patients
- Elevated bradykinin causes vasodilation
- Can be fatal
- Treatment: Stop the ACE-Inhibitor (no duh!)
  ▷ Antihistamines may not work if it's bradykinin medicated
  ▷ Fresh frozen plasma (FFP)
    ◊ Kininase II in FFP breaks down excessive bradykinin
  ▷ Tranexamic acid (TXA)

Recap Post MI Cardiac Meds:

- » ASA indefinitely
- » P2Y$_{12}$ Inhibitor for at least 1 year
- » Beta blocker indefinitely
- » High-dose Statin indefinitely
- » ACE-Inhibitor, ARB, or ARNI if EF ≤ 40%; indefinitely
- » Nitrates if needed for ongoing pain or ischemic issues
  - Fast acting NTG SL
  - Longer acting - Imdur
- » AVOID other NSAIDs!!!! Increases mortality!
  - Increases bleeding and myocardial rupture risk

Post PCI Monitoring & Complications:

- » Access site management
  - Radial artery access site is becoming more common
    - ▷ Easily compressible
    - ▷ Fewer complications
    - ▷ Can spasm – CCB &/or nitrates
    - ▷ May consider direct intra-arterial injection of verapamil or lidocaine
  - Femoral artery access – monitor for bleeding, hematoma, retroperitoneal bleeding
    - ▷ Rare cases, can develop pseudoaneurysms, A/V fistula
    - ▷ Pseudoaneurysm may palpate a pulsating lump, pain & swelling at site
    - ▷ Concern with numbness from nerve compression
    - ▷ Femoral artery ultrasound
- » With retroperitoneal bleeding you may see a "soft" BP that is fluid responsive
  - Tachycardia
    - ▷ May not see if patient received beta blockers
  - Late sign is flank ecchymosis (Grey-Turner's sign)
  - Assess coags
  - Control bleeding
- » Renal function
  - Secondary to IV dye load
  - IV fluids & adequate hydration are key to avoiding Contrast Induced Nephropathy (CIN)
  - See Chapter 8 for additional information on CIN/renal issues

Fibrinolytic Therapy

If Cardiac Catheterization PCI is not available within 90 min, fibrinolytics may be considered.

- » CLOT BUSTING medications
- » Monitor for bleeding!
- » FYI – the patient will still eventually need to go to the cath lab
- » Tenecteplase (TNKase)
  - 5-second bolus
  - No infusion or 2nd bolus
  - Weight-based dosing, no more than 50 mg
  - Less cerebral hemorrhage
- » Activase (rtPA)
  - Bolus followed by infusion

Indications:

- » Pain or symptoms < 6 hours
- » ST elevation > 1 mm in 2 or more contiguous leads
  - Leads that look at the same wall of the heart

Contraindications to fibrinolytics: (higher bleeding risk)

Note: These are the same for embolic stroke or pulmonary embolism

Absolute:

- » Active bleeding
- » Intracranial hemorrhage
- » Known cerebral vascular lesion
- » Ischemic stroke in last 6 mos. (except acute CVA)
- » Malignant intracranial neoplasm
- » Suspected aortic dissection
- » Closed head or facial trauma within 3 mos.
- » A-V Malformation

Relative: (weigh risk vs. benefit)

- » Chronic, severe, poorly tolerated HTN
- » SBP > 180 mm Hg or DBP > 110 mm Hg
  - Lower BP prior to administration
- » Ischemic CVA > 3 mos.
- » Dementia
- » Traumatic or prolonged CPR
- » Major surgery (< 3 weeks)
- » Internal bleeding (within 2 - 4 weeks)
- » Pregnancy
- » Active peptic ulcer disease
- » Current use of anticoagulants

Nursing considerations post fibrinolytic administration:

- » BLEEDING is the most common side effect
  - If bleeding occurs, discontinue all anticoagulation
  - Labs: STAT PT/INR/aPTT & fibrinogen
    ▷ Prolongs PT/aPTT
  - Fibrinogen may be decreased for up to 24 hours
  - Reversal: Cryoprecipitate! FFP & Platelets
  - Think of Cryo as liquid fibrinogen!
- » Frequent neurological assessment (d/t bleeding risk)
  - Intracranial hemorrhage
  - Prepare for STAT head CT scan if there are neuro changes
- » Avoid punctures & central lines for 6 - 12 hours
- » Monitor urine output & BUN/creatinine
- » Avoid invasive devices
- » Avoid compressive devices

Post MI Discharge: Education, Education, Education!

- » Medication adherence
  - Must review medications with patients prior to discharge
  - Utilize teach-back method to evaluate their understanding
- » Minimize ETOH use
  - Must understand interactions with medications
- » Smoking cessation

» Exercise
  • Ideal body weight

» Heart healthy diet
  • Monitor & lower cholesterol & lipids

» Stress reduction

12 Lead ECG

ECG: What do the waves represent?

» P wave: Atrial depolarization

» PR interval: AV conduction time (0.12 – 0.20 sec)

» QRS: Ventricular depolarization (0.06 – 0.10 sec)

» T wave: Ventricular repolarization

» QT interval: Time of ventricular depolarization & repolarization
  • Should always be corrected for rate (QTc)
  • Bazett formula is commonly used
  • Normal QTc - men: 0.35 - 0.45, women: 0.36 - 0.46 sec.

Q-waves—Considered pathologic if:

» Width > 30 ms (0.04 sec)

» Depth ≥ 25% of the height of the R wave

» If present in contiguous leads, indicative of myocardial necrosis

» May or may not develop Q waves with infarcts

12 Lead ECG Summary

Location	ST elevation in lead:	Reciprocal changes in lead: (ST depression)	Artery affected:	Notes:
Anterior/Septal	V_1-V_4	II, III, aVF	LAD/L main	
Lateral	I, aVL, V_5-V_6		L circumflex, L main	
Inferior	II, III, aVF	I, aVL	RCA in 80% L circumflex	Right sided ECG assesses V_2R-V_4R
Right ventricle	V_1, V_2R - V_4R		Proximal RCA	
Posterior	Posterior leads V_{7-9}	V_{1-3}	RCA (90%) L circumflex (10%)	Tall upright R wave in V_1 - V_3

Types of Myocardial Infarctions

Inferior Wall MI

- » Associated with Right Coronary Artery (RCA) occlusion
- » Elevation in leads II, III & aVF
  - Reciprocal changes in leads I & aVL
- » If ST elevation in lead III > lead II, likely RCA occlusion
- » Bedside monitor lead III

Symptoms:

- » Bradycardia
  - AV node ischemia
  - Increased vagal tone from ischemia
  - If symptomatic, can use atropine IV with caution
- » Heart blocks – may need temporary pacer
  - Second degree Type I (Wenckebach)
  - Complete heart block
- » Hypotension

- » N/V
- » Diaphoresis
- » Monitor for signs of right ventricular infarction
- » Papillary muscle rupture
  - New systolic murmur

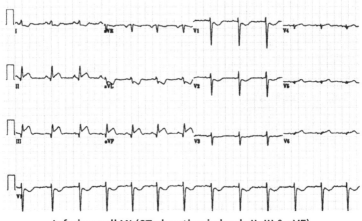

Inferior wall MI (ST elevation in leads II, III & aVF) –
Likely with posterior involvement (ST depression in V_1 & V_2)
Reciprocal changes in leads I & aVL

If right ventricular infarction is suspected, get a right-sided ECG

- » Move precordial leads to right side of chest
- » Key leads are $V_2R - V_4R$
- » If RV infarction will see ST elevation in $V_2R - V_4R$

Right Ventricular Infarction

- » Associated with proximal RCA occlusion & inferior wall MI
- » May see elevation in lead V_1

Symptoms:

- » Tachycardia
- » Hypotension
- » + JVD (with clear lungs)
- » ECHO - the RV is often stunned with poor wall motion; blood backs up to the right side
- » Poor forward flow to the left side of the heart

Treatment:

- » Small crystalloid fluid challenges (maximize preload!)
- » Patients often become preload dependent
- » Use small boluses
- Titrate to effect
- » Next step: + Inotrope
  - Increases contractility
  - Dobutamine

Avoid medications that lower preload:

- » Nitrates, morphine, beta blockers, diuretics
- » RV is stunned & becomes preload dependent

Anterior/Septal Wall MI

- » Changes noted in V_1 - V_4
- » Reciprocal changes in II, III, aVF
- » Loss of R wave progression in the precordial leads (V_1 - V_6)
- » Left anterior descending/left main occlusion

Symptoms:

- » Left ventricular failure (S3 heart sound)
- » Cardiogenic shock
- » Heart block
  - 2nd degree Type 2, 3rd degree
- » Bundle branch block
- » If new loud murmur, suspect ventricular septal rupture or papillary muscle rupture
  - Get an Echocardiogram

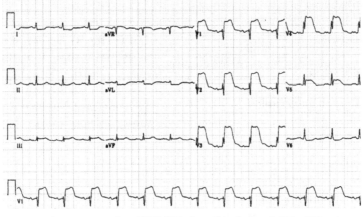

Anteroseptal wall MI (ST elevation in leads V1 – V4)

Conduction defects

Here is a fun & easy way to remember heart blocks!

The Heart Block Poem (original author unknown)

» If the R is far from the P,
then you have a 1st degree

» PR interval gets longer, longer,
longer, the QRS drops, it's
a case of Wenckebach!

» If some R's don't get through,
prepare to PACE that Mobitz II!

» If the R's & P's don't agree,
prepare to PACE that 3rd degree!

First Degree AV Conduction Delay

» Prolonged PR interval

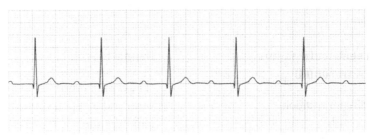

Second Degree AV Block Type 1 (Wenckebach or Mobitz I)

» Progressively longer PR Interval

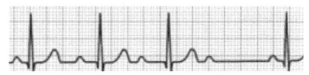

Second Degree AV Block Type 2 (Mobitz II)

» Block occurs below the AV node

» Can progress to CHB

» The PR interval is constant, the QRS complexes (ventricular conduction) are blocked

» If 2:1 block, can be difficult to diagnose
- Prepare to emergently pace!
- Transcutaneous pace first, prepare for transvenous pacing wire insertion

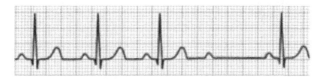

Third Degree AV Block (Complete Heart Block)

» Complete dissociation between the atria & ventricles

» No atrial impulses pass through the AV node

» Ventricles generate their own rhythm

» Ventricular rate is often slow – 20s to 40s

» If the patient is hypotensive or symptomatic:
- Prepare to emergently pace!
- Transcutaneous pace first, then prepare for transvenous pacing wire insertion

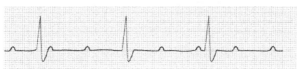

Lateral wall MI

» Changes in V_5, V_6, I, aVL

» Occlusion of the left circumflex or left main

» Can be associated with other MI locations (inferior, anterior)

Posterior Wall MI

» Tall, broad R wave (> 0.04 sec) in V_1 - V_3 & ST depression (reciprocal change)

» Consider a posterior ECG

- ST elevation in posterior leads V_7 - V_9
- Leads follow path around the left chest wall

» Associated with inferior or lateral wall MI

» Occlusion of RCA or left circumflex

- Remember 90% of population is right dominant, the RCA perfuses the posterior wall
- 10% of population is left dominant, the left circumflex perfuses the posterior wall

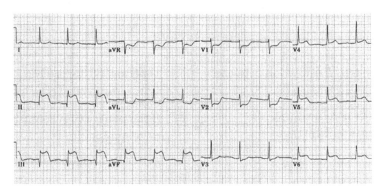

Inferoposterior wall MI (ST elevation in leads II, III, aVF & ST depression in V1, V2 &/or V3)
Reciprocal change: aVL (often Lead I as well)

Complications of Acute Myocardial Infarction

» A quick way to remember complications of myocardial infarctions: (Star Wars fan?!)

Death
Arrhythmias
Regurgitation (valvular)
Tamponade
Heart failure, shock

Valve dysfunction
Aneurysm (ventricular)
Dressler Syndrome
Embolism
Rupture (papillary muscle or ventricular septal)

Pericarditis

» Inflammation of the pericardial sac

» Acute or chronic

» 10 – 15% develops within 2 days to 1 week after myocardial infarction

» Chest pain – sharp, stabbing, or dull & achy
- Pain improved with sitting up & leaning forward
- Left-sided radiation
- Pain worse with cough, positional changes & inspiration

» Pericardial friction rub

» Fever

» ECG changes observed in pericaritis

» Diffuse ST changes
- Depression of the PR interval
- Concave ST segment in limb leads
- A hint it's pericarditis & not a myocardial infarction – ST elevation in leads I & II
  ▷ You wouldn't normally see changes in both leads with ischemia or infarction

Treatment:

» NSAIDs – high dose Ibuprofen
- Colchicine may also be used

» Antibiotic if bacterial, antiviral if virus, antifungal if fungus

Papillary Muscle Rupture

» Clinical signs: associated w/ anterior or inferior wall MI

Clinical symptoms:

» Hemodynamic instability

» New LOUD systolic murmur

» Acute MITRAL REGURGITATION!!!

» Large "v" waves on PAOP waveform

» Often diagnosed by ECHO

Treatment:

» Hemodynamic support

» **Emergent surgical repair/ valve replacement**
- Depends on severity

Ventricular septal rupture

» Associated with septal wall MI

» Oxygen rich blood shunts to the right side of the heart from the left
- Left to right shunting

Symptoms:

» Acute SOB

» S_3 heart sound

» Crackles

» **Holosystolic murmur**

» **PA catheter insertion:**
- Falsely increased C.O. because C.O. reading is derived from the right ventricle (left to right shunting)
- Increased SvO_2 due to left to right shunting
- Large "v" waves on CVP waveform
- Diagnosed by ECHO

Treatment:

- Surgical repair

Cardiogenic Shock
The mortality is about 40 – 50 % when patients develop cardiogenic shock

Clinical signs:

- » S_3, pulmonary edema
- » Tachycardia
- » Arrhythmias
- » Signs of decreased perfusion
- Mottling
- » ↓ UOP
- Oliguria < 0.5 ml/kg/hr

Hemodynamics:

- » Hypotension (MAP < 65 mm Hg)
- » Low C.O. – C.I. < 2 L/min/m²
- » Elevated SVR (afterload)
- » Elevated RAP/CVP (preload)
- » Elevated PAOP (preload)
- » ↓ SvO_2 (< 65%)

Other diagnostics:

- » Cardiac Catheterization if related to ischemia!
  - Percutaneous Coronary Intervention (PCI) for reperfusion
- » ABG – Mixed respiratory & metabolic acidosis; hypoxemia
  - Lactic acidosis due to decreased perfusion & anaerobic metabolism
  - Respiratory acidosis if hypercapnic from pulmonary edema
- » ECHO: ↓ wall motion, reduced ejection fraction
- » Chest x-ray: pulmonary congestion & edema
  - May note opacity due to enlarged pulmonary vasculature
  - Enlarged heart
  - Kerley B lines in lower zones from interstitial edema, usually < 2 cm long
- » BUN/Creatinine – monitor for acute kidney injury
- » Monitor other organs for dysfunction & failure

Supportive Treatment:

- Mechanical circulatory support (i.e. IABP, Impella)
- Vasopressors to support blood pressure
  - Use with caution as they will also increase the SVR & increase the workload of the heart
- \+ Inotrope (i.e. Dobutamine) to improve contractility
- Diuretics (as perfusion allows)
- Afterload reduction / venous vasodilators (i.e. NTG)

Cardiogenic Pulmonary Edema

- Fluid in the alveolus d/t increased alveolar hydrostatic pressures
- Impaired gas exchange, hypercapnia
- Hypoxemia
  - S_3 heart sound
  - Shortness of breath
  - Crackles
  - Pink, frothy sputum
  - Anxiety

Causes:

- Myocardial infarction
- Heart failure
- Hypertensive crisis
- Mitral regurgitation
- Tamponade

Treatment: ↓ preload

- Loop diuretics
- Nitroglycerin
- Morphine
- CPAP or BiPap
  - Oxygen support, may need mechanical ventilation
- Consider + Inotrope (i.e. Dobutamine or Milrinone) to improve contractility

You Can Do It!

Cardiac Medications

Class	Examples	Indications	Effects	Monitor for:	Watch out!
ACE Inhibitors	"prils" —take a "chill-pril"! Class I: Captopril Class II: Enalapril (Vasotec) Ramipril (Altace) Benazepril (Lotensin) Class III: Lisinopril	-CHF/Systolic failure -AMI (EF < 40%) -Anterior wall MI -HTN -Diabetic renal nephropathy	- Vasodilation → preload & afterload - Prevention of myocardial remodeling - Reduce progress of diabetic nephropathy	↓ BP ↑ K⁺ levels	Hypotension Cough Hyperkalemia Angioedema Renal function
Angiotension Receptor Blockers (ARBs)	"sartans" Valsartan, Losartan, Candesartan, Olmesartan, Telmisartan	-HTN -CHF/Systolic failure -Diabetic renal nephropathy -Intolerance of ACE Inhibitors	-Vasodilation -Decreases preload & afterload -Reduces secretion of vasopressin	↓ BP ↑ K⁺ levels	Dizziness Headache Hyperkalemia Caution: MI
Beta Blockers	"olols" **Cardio-selective (blocks B₁):** Bisoprolol, Metoprolol SR, Atenolol, Esmolol (IV), Acebutolol, Nebivolol (Bystolic) **Alpha & Beta Blocking:** Labetalol, Carvedilol (Coreg) **Non-selective (blocks B₁ & B₂):** Propranolol (Inderal), Timolol, Nadolol (Corgard), Sotalol	-HTN -Secondary prevention of MI (only metoprolol tartrate or carvedilol) -Cardiac arrhythmias -Angina -Afib -CHF/Systolic failure	BB = **B**lock the heart **B**reaks on the heart (↓HR) -↓ HR, BP -Negative inotrope, however, decreases myocardial workload → preload -Block endogenous epi & norepi; "stress catecholamine" → morbidity & mortality in HF → arrythmias	↓ HR ↓ BP AV Blocks Heart failure	Bradycardia Hypotension Signs of shock Bronchospasm; Avoid in asthma! Heart block Avoid with cocaine use **Overdose reversal:** Glucagon

Aldosterone Blockers	Spironolactone (Aldactone), Eplerenone (Inspra)	Adjunctive therapy in heart failure	-Diuresis -Blocks Na+ reabsorption → ↓ preload & afterload -In combo with other diuretics, ↓ cardiac workload -K+ sparing diuretic	K+ levels	Hyperkalemia—especially when used with ACE Inhibitors or ARBs
Calcium Channel Blockers (CCBs)	"dipines" used for BP reduction! **Dihydropyridines:** (little effect on contractility or heart rate) Amlodipine, nimodipine, nicardipine (IV), Nifedipine, Felodipine **Benzothiazepine class:** Diltiazem (Cardizem) - HR control **Phenylalkylamine class:** Verapamil (Calan) - HR control	-HTN -To reduce HR -SVT -Afib/flutter -Angina—Prinzmetal's (vasospasm) -Hypertrophic CM -Prevent cerebral artery vasospasm (nimodipine)	-Arterial vasodilation, → ↓ afterload -↓ the force of myocardial contraction -Negative chronotrope -Negative inotrope	→ HR → BP	Heart block Bradycardia Reflexive tachycardia Caution when used with BB **Overdose:** Calcium Chloride & Atropine
Nitrates	Nitroglycerin Isosorbide dinitrate (Isordil), Isosorbide mononitrate (Imdur)	-Angina -Heart failure	-Vasodilation -Venodilation	→ BP Headaches	Hypotension
Hydrazinophthalazine	Hydralazine *Usually prescribed in combo with isosorbide tinitrate, a BB & diuretic in heart failure	-Heart failure -HTN	-Vasodilator → ↓ afterload	→ BP Headaches	Reflexive tachycardia MI/angina

Definitions:
Inotrope—has an effect on contractility, positive inotrope improves contractility, negative inotrope decreases contractility.
Chronotrope—has an effect on heart rate, positive chronotrope increases the heart rate, negative chronotrope decreases the heart rate.

Chapter 3
Hemodynamic Monitoring

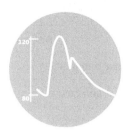

Topics covered in this chapter include:

- Hemodynamic concepts
- Central venous pressure monitoring
- Invasive hemodynamic monitoring (PA Catheter)
- Intra-Aortic Balloon Pump (IABP)
- Monitor hemodynamic status and recognize signs & symptoms of hemodynamic instability
- SvO_2 & $ScvO_2$ monitoring
- Vaopressors, inotropes & vasodilators

Normal Hemodynamic Values

Normal Hemodynamic Values (Know this!!!)	
Cardiac Output (C.O.)	4 – 8 L/min
Cardiac Index (C.I.)	2.5 – 4 L/min/m²
Stroke volume (S.V.)	50 – 100 mL/beat
Stroke volume index	35 – 60 ml/beat/m²
Right ventricular stroke work index (RVSWI)	5 – 10 g/m²/beat
Left ventricular stroke work index (LVSWI)	50 – 62 g/m²/beat
SvO_2	60 – 75%
$ScvO_2$	> 70% (70 – 85%)
Pulmonary artery pressure	25/10 mm Hg
PAOP	8 – 12 mm Hg
RAP/CVP	2 – 6 mm Hg
SVR	900 - 1400 dynes/sec/cm⁵
SVRI	1970 – 2390 dynes/sec/cm⁵/m²
PVR	90 - 250 dynes/sec/cm⁵

An easy way to remember normal intra-cardiac pressures:

Nickel - Dime - Quarter - Dollar!!!
Because we can ALL relate to $$!!!!

A normal RAP/CVP is about a **nickel**
A normal PAOP is about a **dime**
A normal PAP is about a **quarter over a dime**
A normal LV pressure (systolic BP) is about a **dollar!**

You have to know norms! We are so used to looking at abnormal numbers, we forget what norms are! (OR, maybe you rarely see PA catheters anymore...the struggle is real!)

Hemodynamic Concepts

Cardiac output (C.O.):

» Amount of blood ejected by the ventricles per minute

» C.O. = Heart rate (HR) x Stroke volume (SV)

- Normal C.O. = 4 - 8 L/min
- Normal Cardiac Index (C.I.) = 2.5 – 4.0 L/min/m²
- Cardiac Index = C.O. divided by Body Surface Area (BSA)

» Can be measured:
- Pulmonary artery catheter
- Echocardiogram
- Indirectly via functional hemodynamics
- Non-invasive methods (Bioreactance & continuous digit C.O.)
- Fick equation

» C.O. may be normal when the patient is tachycardic with lower SV
- In low output states, patients compensate with tachycardia

Stroke volume (SV):

» Normal is 50 - 100 mL/beat

» Normal stroke volume index (SVI) = 35 – 60 ml/beat/m²

» The amount of blood ejected with each beat

» SV = End diastolic volume (EDV) – End systolic volume (ESV)

- Typical EDV = 120 ml
  ▷ Amount of blood in the heart at the end of diastole
- Typical ESV = 50 ml
  ▷ Amount of blood in the ventricles at the end of ejection/systole

» Three measures contribute to SV:
- Preload
  ▷ Myocardial fiber length at the end of diastole
- Afterload
  ▷ Resistance the heart has to eject against during systole
- Contractility
  ▷ Strength of myofibril contraction

Preload

- » Defined as the stretching of cardiac myocytes prior to ejection

- » Volume concept, measured as pressure (with caution)

- » Indirectly measured on the <u>right side</u>:
  - Right Atrial Pressure (RAP)
  - Central Venous Pressure (CVP)
  - Normal 2 – 6 mm Hg

  Note: CVP & RAP are essentially the same. CVP is obtained from the distal port of a central line, RAP from a PA Catheter

- » **End diastole**
  - Volume of blood filling the ventricle during diastole

- » Indirectly measured on the <u>left side</u>:
  - Pulmonary Artery Occlusive Pressure (PAOP)
  - Normal 8 – 12 mm Hg
  - Reflective of left atrial pressure
  - PAOP is always lower than the PA diastolic

Conditions causing an increase in preload:

- » Heart failure
- » Hypervolemia
- » Cardiogenic shock
- » RV failure (↑ CVP)
- » Ventricular septal defect (VSD) (↑ CVP)
- » Pulmonary hypertension (↑ CVP)

- » Tricuspid stenosis (↑ CVP)
- » Mitral stenosis (↑ PAOP)
- » Pericardial tamponade (↑ CVP & PAOP)
- » Increasing PEEP on the ventilator (↑ intrathoracic chest pressure)
  - Also decreases, see next page
- » IV fluids (at least that's usually the goal!)

Conditions causing a decrease in preload:

- » Hypovolemia for whatever reason (bleeding)
- » Diuretics
- » Veno/vasodilation
- » Decreased venous return
- » After the administration of morphine, NTG or beta blockers!
- » Increasing PEEP on the ventilator
  - ↓ venous return from IVC collapse

Afterload (Systemic Vascular Resistance)

- » Defined as the pressure or resistance the ventricles must overcome to eject blood
- » Pulmonary vascular resistance (PVR)
  - Right ventricular afterload
  - Normal 90 - 250 dynes/sec/cm^5
- » Systemic vascular resistance (SVR)
  - Left ventricular afterload
  - Normal 900 - 1400 dynes/sec/cm^5
  - Formula = $\frac{MAP - CVP(80)}{C.O.}$

Conditions causing an increase in afterload:

- » Cardiogenic shock
- » Hypovolemic shock
- » Bleeding
- » Heart failure
- » Cardiac tamponade
- » Use of vasopressors (i.e. epinephrine, norepinephrine)
- » Think **vasoconstriction!**

Conditions causing a decrease in afterload:

- » Distributive Shock
- » Septic shock (warm stage)
- » Anaphylactic shock
- » Spinal/neurogenic shock
- » Vasodilators (i.e. Nitroglycerin, Nipride)
- » Vasoplegic Shock
- » Milrinone, Dobutamine
- » Think **vasodilation!**

Contractility

- » Force of ventricular ejection
- » Difficult to measure
- » Influenced by changes in preload & afterload
- » "Inotrope" +/-
  - + inotropes will increase contractility (i.e. Dobutamine)
  - − inotropes will decrease contractility (i.e. beta blockers)

Other factors affecting contractility:

- » STEMI (↓)
- » Sepsis (↑ or ↓)
- » Inadequate stretch (↓)
- » Severe hypoxia (↓)
- » ↑ Resistance
  - Increased SVR/afterload (↓)
- » ↑ H^+ (acidosis) (↓)
- » Hypercapnia/ ↑ CO_2 (↓)

SvO_2/$ScvO_2$:

- » True mixed venous O_2 saturation
- » Measures relationship between oxygen delivery & consumption
- » Normal SvO_2 60 – 75%
  - Measured with a pulmonary artery catheter
- » $ScvO_2$ 70% - 85%
  - Surrogate of mixed venous – central venous
  - Runs about 5 – 8% higher than SvO_2
- » If you cannot continuously monitor $ScvO_2$:
  - Draw sample from distal tip of TLC/PICC (thorax) positioned in the superior vena cava
- » Normal oxygen extraction ratio (O_2ER) = 25 – 30%
- » In other words, we normally extract 25 – 30% of oxygen to the tissues & 70 – 75% comes back to the heart & is measured via SvO_2 or $ScvO_2$

If the SvO$_2$ or ScvO$_2$ is low, ask yourself if it is a delivery or consumption problem!

- » DO$_2$ (O$_2$ delivery) is affected by 3 physiologic parameters:
  - "The Pump"
    - ▷ Is the cardiac output adequate?
  - "The Lungs"
    - ▷ Is the oxygenation adequate? Excessive metabolic demands?
  - "The Hemoglobin"
    - ▷ Is there adequate O$_2$ carrying capacity?

- » VO$_2$ (↑ O$_2$ consumption) is affected by:
  - Increased work of breathing
  - Shivering
  - Fever
  - Infection
  - Agitation
  - Turning/mobility
  - Nursing care

The Pulmonary Artery Catheter (PAC)

» a.k.a. "Swan-Ganz" catheter

Contraindications to PA Catheter insertion:

- » Tricuspid or pulmonic prosthetic valve
- » Right heart mass (thrombus or tumor)
- » Tricuspid or pulmonic valve endocarditis
- » Left BBB

Direct measurements from the PAC:

- » Right atrial pressure (RAP/CVP)
- » Pulmonary artery pressures (PAS/PAD)
- » Pulmonary artery occlusive pressure (PAOP)
- » C.O.
- » SvO$_2$

Calculated measurements:

- SV/SVI
- C.I.
- SVR
- PVR
- DO_2

Guidelines for any transduced pressure waveform:

- **Level at the phlebostatic axis**
  - 4th ICS & ½ AP diameter (level of left atrium)
  - Eliminates effects of hydrostatic forces on the observed hemodynamic
  - Ensure air-fluid interface of the transducer is leveled before zeroing &/or obtaining pressure readings

- **Over-damped waveform:**
  - Sluggish, artificially rounded & blunted appearance
  - SBP erroneously low; DBP erroneously high
  - Causes: large air bubbles in system, compliant tubing, loose/open connections, and low fluid level in flush bag

- 0 - 60° HOB elevation
- **Dynamic response testing (a.k.a square wave test)**
  - Fast flush – should see 1 – 3 oscillatory waves following flush
  - Optimal test ensures the line is reliable

- **Under-Damped waveform:**
  - Over responsive, exaggerated, artificially spiked waveform
  - SBP erroneously high; DBP erroneously low
  - Causes: small air bubbles, too long of tubing, defective transducer

Rules for measuring HD waveforms:

- **Measure at end-expiration**
- **Interpret the CVP & PAOP at the mean of the a – c wave**
- **Ensure transducer is leveled at the phlebostatic axis**
- **Ensure line is reliable (dynamic response test)**

RAP/CVP & PAOP waveforms consist of:

- » a wave—upstroke of atrial systole
  - Produced after atrial depolarization; (after PR interval)
- » c wave—often not visible
  - Closure of the tricuspid valve for CVP, mitral valve for PAOP
- » v wave—atrial diastole when tricuspid valve is closed
  - Produced after ventricular depolarization; QSR complex
- » Read the mean of the "a" & "c" wave <u>or</u>
  - Z-point method: read at the end of QRS complex
  - Z-point is the method used when patients are in Afib or junctional rhythms
- » Remember! Mechanical events (contraction) follow electrical events (depolarization)
  - Lightening happens before the thunder!

Pulmonary artery pressure (PAP)

- » Normal PA pressure = 25/10 mm Hg
  - Quarter over a dime

Causes of elevated systolic (PAS):

- » Pulmonary embolism
- » COPD
- » ARDS
- » Hypoxia
- » Pulmonary HTN
- » Cor pulmonale

Causes of elevated diastolic (PAD):

- » Left ventricular failure
- » Mitral valve dysfunction
- » Cardiac tamponade

PA diastolic (PAD) is reflective of LVEDP except with:

- » Mitral valve dysfunction
- » Pulmonary HTN
- » Right BBB
- » Aortic insufficiency
- » Pulmonic insufficiency
- » Decreased LV compliance

PAOP "Wedge" pressure

- » Normal 8 - 12 mm Hg
  - About a dime
- » Preload indicator
- » Estimates left atrial filling pressures
- » PAOP should be < PAD
- » Assumes pressure & volume are directly proportional
  - However, that is only in a normally compliant ventricle!
  - Disproportionate increase in pressure w/ an increase in volume
  - Compliance is a change in pressure for a given change in volume

Some safety tips for PAOP:

- » Inject air into the balloon port slowly & stop when the waveform changes
- » Never inject more than 1.5 ml of air
- » Stop inflating the balloon if resistance is met
- » Inflate < 15 seconds
- » Allow air to passively exit
- » If PA waveform does not change, this may a sign of:
  - Balloon rupture
  - Tip of PA is in the RV or in PA

PAOP waveform consists of:

- » a wave = atrial contraction (after QRS)
- » c wave = mitral valve closure (often not visible)
- » v wave – atrial filling (after T wave)

General PAOP guidelines:

Elevated in:

- » Mitral stenosis
- » Mitral insufficiency
- » Left ventricular failure
- » Fluid/volume overload
- » Cardiac tamponade
- » Constrictive pericarditis
- » High levels of PEEP

Lung zones

» PA Cath tip must be placed in Zone 3
» Signs in Zone 1 or 2:
- Damped PAOP waveform
- PAOP > PAD
- Absence of a & v waves

Causes of large "v" waves (CVP or PAOP)

» Mitral regurgitation (PAOP)
» Tricuspid regurgitation (CVP)
» Fluid overload (Could be either – primarily PAOP)
» Ventricular septal rupture (CVP)

Shock Hemodynamics

Types of Shock	CO/CI	Preload: CVP	Preload: PAOP	Afterload: SVR	Treatment
Cardiogenic (left ventricular)	Decreased	Increased or normal	Increased	Increased	+ Inotropes, Afterload reduction, Pressors
Cardiogenic (right ventricular)	Decreased	Increased	Normal or decreased	Increased	Fluids, + inotropes, Pulm vasod.
Obstructive (Tamponade)	Decreased	Increased	Increased	Increased	Pericardio-centesis or OR
Hypovolemic/ Hemorrhage	Decreased	Decreased	Decreased	Increased	Fluids or blood
Vasodilatory / Septic	Increased or normal	Decreased or normal	Decreased or normal	Decreased	Fluid, Vasopressors!

Intra-Aortic Balloon Counterpulsation IABC/IABP

- Used in cardiogenic shock & decompensated heart failure
- Balloon <u>inflates</u> at the onset of <u>diastole</u>
  - Inflates at the dicrotic notch
  - Dicrotic notch signifies closure of the aortic valve
  - Coronary arteries are perfused during diastole
- Balloon <u>deflates</u> immediately before <u>systole</u>
  - Afterload or resistance to ejection is reduced
- Femoral artery insertion is common
  - Can also insert brachial or transthoracic
  - Monitor pulses distal to the insertion site

Benefits of IABP:

- Increased coronary artery perfusion
- Increased perfusion to organs
- Increased O_2 supply
- Increased O_2 supply
- Decreased O_2 demand
- Decreased afterload

Position of IABP catheter:

- 2nd to 3rd ICS
  - Inferior to subclavian artery
  - Superior to renal artery
- Palpate left radial pulse
  - If unable to palpate, catheter is positioned too high
- Monitor urine output closely
  - If dropping, catheter may be positioned too low

Contraindications to IABP:

- Aortic insufficiency
- Aortic aneurysm
- Aortic calcifications (can cause balloon rupture)

Complications of IABP:

- » Limb ischemia
- » Incorrect timing
- » Malposition
- » Renal artery occlusion (if positioned too low)
- » Infection
- » Balloon rupture
- » Bleeding

Pharmacologic Action & Target – Catecholamine Vasopressors & Inotropes

Drug	Alpha	Beta$_1$	Beta$_2$
Vasopressors			
Phenylephrine	++++	-	-
Norepinephrine	++++	++	-
Epinephrine	++++	++++	++
Dopamine (dose dependent)	++ < 5 mcg/kg/min	++++ < 10 mcg/kg/min	+
	+++ > 10 mcg/kg/min		
Inotrope			
Dobutamine (+ inotrope)	+	++++	++

Adrenergic receptors:

- » Alpha—located in blood vessels
- » Beta$_1$— located on the heart
- » Beta$_2$— located in the bronchial & vascular smooth muscle

Vasopressors: Used to increase blood pressure!

Norepinephrine (Levophed)

- Effect: ↑ BP, ↑ SVR, ↑ C.O. (mild increase)
- Mostly alpha & some beta$_1$

Dosing:

- 0.5 – 30 mcg/min
- Half-life is about 2 minutes
- Monitor closely for extravasation

Adverse Effects:

- Bradycardia, dysrhythmias, HTN, renal artery vasoconstriction

Epinephrine (Adrenalin)

- Effect: ↑ BP, ↑ HR, ↑ SVR, ↑ C.O.
- Also going to increase oxygen consumption (VO$_2$)
- Alpha, beta$_1$, some beta$_2$

Dosing:

- 1 - 10 mcg/min – titrate to effect
- Always try to use the lowest dose possible

Adverse effects:

- HTN, myocardial ischemia, increased oxygen consumption, tachycardia, dysrhythmias, chest pain
- Monitor closely for extravasation – can cause tissue necrosis
- Watch for hyperglycemia
- May see lactate levels increase with use, especially in sepsis

Phenylephrine (Neo-Synephrine)

- » Effect: ↑ BP, ↑ SVR
- » Pure alpha receptor stimulant
- » Less vasoconstriction than norepinephrine
- » No effect on HR to produce tachycardia

Dosing:

- » 2 - 10 mcg/kg/min
  - 10 – 180 mcg/min
- » Half-life is about 2.5 to 3 min

Adverse effects:

- » Reflex bradycardia, dysrhythmias, HTN, chest pain
- » Monitor for extravasation

Dopamine (Inotropin)

- » Effect: ↑ HR, ↑ BP, ↑ SVR, ↑ C.O. (dose dependent)
- » Classified as a catecholamine
- » Acts on the SNS
- » Positive inotropic effects
- » Stimulates beta$_1$ & some beta$_2$, alpha
- » Watch for tachyarrhythmias & ventricular ectopy
- » Monitor closely for extravasation – can cause tissue necrosis

Dosing:

- » 0.5 - 3 mcg/kg/min – dopaminergic receptors
  - May see in ↑ BP
- » 3 - 10 mcg/kg/min – beta effects
  - ↑ BP & CO
- » > 10 mcg/kg/min – alpha effects
  - ↑ BP
- » Max usually 20 mcg/kg/min
- » Onset of action is about 5 minutes
- » Half-life is about 2 minutes

Effects:

- » Low doses – increased urine output
- » Higher doses – *tachycardia*, increased SVR, increased workload of heart (d/t vasoconstriction), myocardial ischemia, renal ischemia, atrial & ventricular arrhythmias
- » NOTE: It is no longer recommended to use "renal dose Dopamine"!
- » Not used much because of tachycardia & arrhythmias

Vasopressin (Pitressin)

- » Effect: ↑BP, ↑SVR
- » Natural anti-diuretic hormone (ADH)
- » 2nd line vasopressor in Sepsis
- » Use in caution in patients with CAD
- » Also given for GI Bleeding & Diabetes Insipidus

Dosing:

- » 0.01 – 0.1 units/min
- » Usually start at 0.03 units/min
- » Half-life 10 – 20 min

Vasopressor extravasations:

Phentolamine (Regitine)

- » Alpha$_1$ blocker
- » Used for vasopressor or Dilantin extravasation
  - Also used for treatment of hypertension
- » Phentolamine mesylate 5 – 10 mg diluted in 10 – 15 ml of saline
- » Inject around infiltrated site
- » Prevents necrosis & sloughing of tissue
- » Limits extravasation ischemia
- » Also consider warm compresses
- » Topical nitroglycerin paste can also be used

Positive Inotropes

- » Used to improve cardiac output & contractility

Dobutamine (Dobutrex)

- » Effect: ↑ C.O., ↑ HR, ↓ SVR, ↓ PAOP
- » Stimulates beta receptors, beta$_1$ (some alpha)
- » Also used in cardiac surgery & septic shock

Dosing:

- » 2 – 20 mcg/kg/min IV (up to 40 mcg/kg/min)
- » Onset 1 - 2 minutes, up to 10 min.
- » Plasma half-life is 2 minutes, so just decrease or discontinue hypotensive
- » Monitor for: tachycardia, hypo or hypertension, ectopy, hypokalemia
- » May develop tolerance after a few days

Milrinone (Primacor)

- » Effects: ↑ C.O., ↓ PAOP & SVR, no change in HR
- » Phosphodiesterase (PDE) inhibitor
  - Inhibits the degradation of cyclic AMP in cardiac & smooth muscle
  - Increases calcium influx into the cells
- » Used mostly in exacerbated heart failure
- » Vasodilatory effects – watch for hypotension!
- » Often called an "Inodilator"

Dosing:

- » Bolus 50 mcg/kg over 10 min.
  - Bolus rarely given
- » Maintenance: 0.375 – 0.75 mcg/kg/min
  - Reduce dose in renal failure
- » Long half-life – about 2.5 hours!!!!
- » Hepatic clearance

Adverse effects:

- » Ventricular irritability – PVCs, hypotension, angina
- » Correct hypokalemia & hypovolemia before administering!
- » Avoid in patients with severe valve disease or acute MI
- » Dilates venous vasculature
  - ↓ Preload
  - Has some arterial effect
    - ▷ Afterload reducer

Vasodilators

» Used to decrease SVR & resistance or decrease BP

Nitroprusside (Nipride)

» Antihypertensive of nitrate origin

» AFTERLOAD reducer!

» Also reduces preload

Dosing:

» 0.1 – 8 mcg/kg/min

» Arterial line preferred if titrating

Adverse effects:

» Hypotension
- Assess BP Q 1 - 2 min until BP is stabilized

» Hypoxia (from intrapulmonary shunt)

» Increased HR
- Stimulation of baroreceptors

» Thiocyanate toxicity (esp. if given > 72 hrs.), monitor levels

» Methemoglobinemia (Hgb can get converted)

» Do not use in hypotension, hypovolemia, aortic stenosis

Nitroglycerin (Tridil)

» Potent peripheral vasodilator

» Used to treat: angina, HF, HTN

» Dilates arterial & venous vasculature
- Preload & afterload reducer!

Dosing:

» 5 mcg/min up to 200 mcg/min

» Can titrate pretty quickly – every 5 to 10 minutes

Adverse effects:

» Hypotension, bradycardia, dizziness, hypovolemia, headache, reflexive tachycardia, N/V

» Do not use in hypotension, hypovolemia, aortic stenosis, ICP issues, constrictive pericarditis

» In some people NTG doesn't have much effect on the BP

Vasopressors & Positive Inotropes: How they affect hemodynamics

Medication	HR	MAP	C.O.	SVR	PAOP
Vasopressors					
Norepinephrine	-	↑↑↑	↑	↑↑↑	↑/-
Epinephrine	↑↑↑	↑↑↑	↑↑↑	↑↑↑	↑/-
Dopamine	↑↑	↑↑	↑↑	↑↑	↓
Phenylephrine	-	↑↑↑	-	↑↑↑	↑/-
Vasopressin	-	↑↑	-	↑↑↑	↑/-
Positive inotropes					
Dobutamine	↑↑↑	↑/↓	↑↑↑	↓/-	↓
Milrinone	-	↑/↓	↑↑↑	↓	↓
Vasodilators					
Nitroglycerin	-	↓	↑/-	↓	↓↓
Nitroprusside	-	↓↓↓	↑↑	↓↓↓	↓↓
Nicardipine	-	↓↓	↑/-	↓↓	↓/-
Esmolol	↓	↓	↓/-	↓	↓/-

↑ = little effect, ↑↑ = moderate, ↑↑↑ = major, (-) = not much

See "Other Cardiac Issues & Complications" chapter for additional anti-hypertensive (vasodilator) medications.

Chapter 4
Heart Failure & Cardiomyopathies

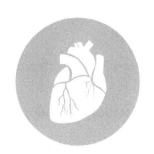

Topics covered in this chapter include:

- Acute exacerbation
- HFrEF, HFpEF, HFmEF
- Etiology of heart failure – left, right, diastolic, systolic
- Cardiomyopathy – dilated, hypertrophic, restrictive
- Stress-induced (Takotsubo)

Heart Failure

2 types:

1. Heart Failure with preserved EF (HFpEF)

Diastolic Heart Failure

- Ejection Fraction ≥ 50%
- HFmEF=EF 41 – 49%
- Stiff non-compliant ventricle & left ventricular hypertrophy (LVH)
- Usually history of hypertension
- Treatment focuses on controlling BP
- Manage symptoms with diuretics if needed

2. Heart Failure with reduced EF (HFrEF)

Systolic Heart Failure

- Ejection Fraction ≤ 40%
- AKA: "Congestive Heart Failure"
- Acute Decompensated HF
- ↑preload, ↑afterload, ↓contractility

"...complex clinical syndrome (collection of symptoms) that results from any structural or functional impairment of ventricular filling or ejection of blood" (AHA definition)

Risk factors for developing heart failure:

- **Coronary artery disease/MI**
  - 8 – 10 times increased risk (HFrEF)
- **Hypertension**
  - 2 – 3 times increased risk (HFpEF)
- **Diabetes**
  - 2 – 5 times increased risk (HFrEF or HFpEF)
  - Metabolic syndrome
- **Valvular disease**
  - (HFrEF or HFpEF)

Other reasons for heart failure:

» Obesity
- Every 1 kg/m² increase in BMI is associated with 5% increased risk in men, 7% in women

» Chronic alcoholism

» Pregnancy

» Family history

» Takotsubo cardiomyopathy

» Drugs

- Cocaine, chemo, anabolic steroids

» Connective tissue disorders
- Lupus, sarcoidosis, scleroderma, amyloidosis

» Tachycardia induced CM

» Idiopathic
- Means we don't know why!

Metabolic Syndrome

» Estimated 25% of the U.S. population have it
- 40% incidence age > 60

» High risk for developing CV disease, stroke & diabetes

"The Deadly Quartet" - Any 2 of the following:

» Dyslipidemia
- Elevated triglycerides > 150 mg/dL
- Low HDL < 40 in males, < 50 in female

» Hypertension
- SBP > 130 or DBP > 85

» Hyperglycemia
- Fasting blood glucose > 100 or diagnosed Type 2 DM

» Abdominal obesity
- Waistline > 40 inches men, > 35 inches women

Ventricular failure – left vs. right side

Left sided failure: blood backs up to the lungs

» Tachypnea

» Tachycardia

» S$_3$ heart sound – ventricular gallop

» Mitral regurgitation

» Displaced point of maximal impulse (PMI)

» Crackles

» Cough, frothy sputum

» ↑ PA pressures

» ↑ PAOP – elevated "v" waves on PAOP

» ↓ C.O./C.I.

» ↑ afterload (SVR)

Wet lungs

Right sided failure: blood backs up to the venous periphery

» JVD

» Hepatojugular reflux

» Peripheral edema

» Hepatomegaly

» Anorexia, N/V

» Bendopnea

» Ascites

» Tricuspid regurgitation

» ↑ CVP – elevated "v" wave on CVP

» ↑ Liver enzymes

» Increased PVR

Clear lungs
(in isolated right failure)

With reduced EF & heart failure, patients may start with left ventricular failure, but the right side fails over time.

Assessment in heart failure:

PMI (Point of maximum impulse)

- » Normally palpated at the 5th ICS, MCL @ the apex
- » Displaced in HF
  - Downward & to the left

Causes of PMI shifting:

- » Left ventricular hypertrophy
- » Heart failure
- » Right pneumothorax
- » Right pleural effusion

Measuring Jugular Venous Distention (JVD)

- » Supine position, HOB 30°
- » Turn head slightly to left – note: the right jugular is aligned directly with the right atrium
- » Observe for pulsations
- » Note highest point
- » Measure distance between the pulsation and sternal angle
- » 4 cm above sternal angle is normal

Heart Failure Diagnostics

- » ECHO
  - Assess ejection fraction, wall motion, chamber size
- » Trans-Esophageal Echo (TEE) – assess heart function and presence of thrombus
- » Brain Natriuretic Peptide (BNP) level – will be elevated
  - Also use NT-proBNP
  - Elevated with over stretch of ventricle
- » 12 Lead ECG – assess for ischemia, BBB, atrial enlargement, valvular regurg
- » Chest radiograph – assess for congestion & fluid overload
- » Angiogram indicated for ischemia
- » Myocardial biopsy
  - For restrictive CM

HFrEF - Reduced EF Systolic Heart Failure

- » Also called "Dilated Cardiomyopathy"
- » Damage to myofibrils
- » Poor forward flow of blood
- » ↑ preload & afterload
- » Systolic & diastolic dysfunction
- » Elevated BNP Levels

BNP Levels

- » Hormone/peptide secreted by ventricles in response to stretch
- » Allows for rapid diagnosis of heart failure

> **Levels:**
>
> < 100 no heart failure
>
> ~ 100 - 300 heart failure is present
>
> > 300 mild heart failure
>
> > 600 moderate heart failure
>
> > 900 severe heart failure
>
> Reference: Cleveland Clinic originally validated BNP in the Breathing Not Properly study (Level > 100 pg/mL 90% sensitivity 76% specificity to predict HF)

Heart failure (HFrEF) treatment strategies

Goal: Blunt the Sympathetic Nervous System (SNS), Renin Angiotensin Aldosterone System (RAAS), Aldosterone & Neprilysin

Cardiomyopathy management: Optimize heart function

- » Reduce preload
- » Reduce afterload
- » Improve contractility – forward flow of blood

Heart Failure & Cardiomyopathies

General Medical management

» 1st line: ACE Inhibitor ("prils")
OR
Angiotensin Receptor Blocker ARB ("sartans")
OR
Angiotensin Receptor Blocker/ Neprilysin Inhibitor (ARNI)

- Entresto (sacubitril/valsartan)

» Beta-blocker OR Alpha/beta blocker

- Carvedilol
- Metoprolol succinate
- Bisoprolol
- Goal to keep HR < 80

» SGLT-2 Inhibitor

- Esp. beneficial in patients with Type 2 Diabetes
- Added in Stage C or D heart failure once on ACE-I, ARB or ARNI, BB & aldosterone antagonist

» Aldosterone antagonist (i.e. spironolactone, eplerenone)

» Hydralazine (afterload reducer) & isosorbide dinitrate (preload reducer) combo

- Preload & afterload reducers

» Diuretics (usually loop)

» Cardiac glycosides (i.e. digoxin)

- Not a first line agent

FYI - new-ish Heart Failure Medication

» Entresto™ (sacubitril/valsartan)

» Class: ARB/Neprilysin inhibitor (ARNI)

» Indicated to reduce the risk of cardiovascular death and hospitalization for heart failure (HF) in patients with chronic heart failure (CHF) (NYHA class II-IV) & reduced ejection fraction

» Recommended starting dose: 49 mg/51 mg PO BID

» Target maintenance dose: After 2 - 4 weeks, double the dose to the target maintenance dose of 97 mg/103 mg PO BID as tolerated

» 20% mortality reduction compared to Enalapril

> *In hemodynamically stable, but somewhat hypotensive HF patients, when would you hold medications?*
>
> **This is my favorite quote I heard at an AHA Conference:**
> "There is a difference between hypotension & symptomatic hypotension... in heart failure, this is important! Know the difference!"
>
> **GIVE THE MEDS!!!**
>
> ...only hold for <u>symptomatic</u> hypotension

Acute decompensated HF escalated management:

- Positive inotropes - Dobutamine or Milrinone
  - Used to improve cardiac output & contractility
  - Also have vasodilatory effects – reduces afterload
- Loop diuretics
  - Remove fluid
- Afterload reduce with vasodilators

- Nitroglycerin (Tridil)
  - ↓ preload
  - Mild ↓ afterload
- Hold beta blockers!
  - Because of negative inotropic effects!
- CPAP or BiPAP if needed

Dobutamine (Dobutrex)

- Effect: ↑ C.O., ↑ HR, ↓ SVR, ↓ PAOP
- Stimulates beta receptors, Beta$_1$ (some alpha)

- Also used in cardiac surgery & septic shock

Dosing:

- 2 – 20 mcg/kg/min IV (up to 40 mcg/kg/min)

- Onset 1 - 2 minutes, up to 10 min.

- » Plasma half-life 2 minutes
  - If hypotensive, decrease the dose or discontinue
- » Monitor for: tachycardia, hypo/hypertension, ectopy, hypokalemia
- » May develop tolerance after a few days

Milrinone (Primacor)

- » Effects: ↑C.O., ↓PAOP & SVR, no change in HR
- » Phosphodiesterase (PDE) inhibitor
  - Inhibits the degradation of cyclic AMP in cardiac & smooth muscle
  - Increases calcium influx into the cells
- » Used mostly in exacerbated heart failure
- » Vasodilatory effects – watch for hypotension!
  - Called an "inodilator"

Dosing:

- » May bolus 50 mcg/kg over 10 min.
- » Maintenance: 0.375 – 0.75 mcg/kg/min
  - Reduce in renal failure
- » Long half-life – about 2.5 hours!!!!
- » Hepatic clearance

Adverse effects:

- » Hypotension
- » Ventricular irritability – PVCs
- » Angina
- » Correct hypokalemia & hypovolemia before administration!
- » Avoid in patients with severe valve disease or acute MI

Vasodilators

Used in heart failure to decrease the afterload & preload

Nitroprusside (Nipride)

- Antihypertensive of nitrate origin
- Arterial line preferred if titrating for blood pressure
- Potent vasodilator and AFTERLOAD reducer!
- Also reduces preload

Dosing:

- 0.1 – 8 mcg/kg/min
- Half-life 2 min

Adverse effects:

- Hypotension
  - Assess BP Q 1 - 2 min until BP is stabilized
  - Ask for an art line!
- Hypoxia (from intrapulmonary shunt)
- Increased HR (stimulation of baroreceptors)
- Thiocyanate poisoning
  - esp. if given > 72 hrs.
  - check level
- Methemoglobinemia (Hgb can get converted)
- Do not use in hypotension, hypovolemia, aortic stenosis

Nitroglycerin (Tridil)

- » Potent peripheral vasodilator
- » Dilates arterial & venous vasculature
- » Preload & afterload reducer!
- » Used to treat: angina, HF, HTN

Dosing:

- » 5 mcg/min up to 200 mcg/min
- » Can titrate pretty quickly – every 5 to 10 minutes

Adverse effects:

- » Hypotension, bradycardia, dizziness, hypovolemia, headache, reflexive tachycardia, N/V
- » In some people NTG doesn't have much effect on the BP
- » Do not use in hypotension, hypovolemia, aortic stenosis, ICP issues, constrictive pericarditis

Heart Failure Discharge Education

- » Medication adherence
- » Activity
- » Sodium restricted diet
  - Fluid restriction debatable; fluid restrict if hyponatremic, Na^+ restrict if pulmonary congestion
  - Na^+ is the nemesis of heart failure
- » Daily weight
- » Smoking cessation
- » Limit alcohol intake
- » Weight loss is applicable
- » Prevent infection – flu & pneumococcal vaccines

Long term heart failure options

- » Cardiac Resynchronization Therapy (CRT) if patient has a BBB

- » Cardiac Assist Devices (i.e. IABP, Impella - short term) or VAD (long term)

- » Cardiac transplant

- » + Inotropes (i.e. Dobutamine or Milrinone) - palliative

- » CardioMEMS sensor
  - Trends PA pressures at home

Cardiac Resynchronization Therapy (CRT)

- » Biventricular Pacemaker

- » Indicated for EF < 35% with a QRS duration > 0.12 sec

- » Bi-ventricular pacing results in shortened QRS duration & better ventricular synchrony

Benefits:

- » Synchronized ventricular contraction

- » Increased EF/C.O.

- » Symptom improvement

- » Compliment medical therapy

- » Improve quality of life

- » Gives hope to those who are suffering with moderate to severe heart failure

- » Reduced mortality

Ventricular Assist Device (VAD)

- » Left (LVAD), right (RVAD) or both (BiVAD)

- » **Short term VAD**
  - Bridge to transplant

- » **Long term VAD**
  - Destination therapy
  - LVAD
  - Palliative to give the patient extra time

Cardiac transplantation

- » Vagal nerve is severed
- » Atropine will not work if bradycardia develops – need to pace!
- » Immunosuppression to prevent rejection
- » Prone to infections

Hypertrophic Cardiomyopathy (HCM)

Physiologic changes:

- » Thickened interventricular septum
  - The septum is normally about 6 – 10 mm in width
  - Often > 15 – 20 mm in width in HCM
  - Can lead to aortic outflow tract obstruction
- » Diastolic dysfunction & left ventricular hypertrophy
- » Decreased ventricular compliance
- » Assessment: S_4, murmur, displaced PMI
- » May present with sudden cardiac death
- » Genetic—caused by a mutation in one of several sarcomere genes
- » Anti-arrhythmics if indicated
  - Amiodarone
  - Disopyramide (Norpace)

Diagnostics:

- » Echocardiogram
  - Assess septum & presence of LVH
- » 12 Lead ECG
  - Signs of LVH
- » Cardiac MRI
- » Stress test

Treatment:

- » Beta blockers &/or calcium channel blockers
  - Goal: SLOW the heart to prolong diastole & filling time!
- » Avoid inotropes!!!
  - Digoxin/dobutamine
- » Implantable Cardioverter Defibrillator (ICD) - prevent sudden cardiac death & ventricular arrhythmias

- » Reduce the septum:
  - Percutaneous transluminal septal myocardial ablation (PTSMA)
  - Alcohol ablation of the septum
    - ▷ Monitor for heart attack
  - Septal Myomectomy
    - ▷ Remove septal muscle contributing to aortic outflow obstruction
    - ▷ Considered when symptoms don't improve with meds

Takotsubo Cardiomyopathy

- » Also called "Broken Heart Syndrome" or "Stress Induced Cardiomyopathy"
- » Result of severe emotional or physical stress
- » Possibly the result of a surge in stress hormones (i.e. adrenaline)

- » Weakening & ballooning of the left ventricle
- » Happens almost exclusively in women over age 55 (~90%)
- » Often resolves within one month

Symptoms:

- » Chest pain
- » SOB
- » Can see ST elevations on the 12 Lead ECG

- » Cardiac cath is often clean
- » About 30% go into cardiogenic shock
  - Decreased EF predicts shock

Treatment:

- » Short term heart failure meds:
  - ACE Inhibitor or ARB
  - Beta blocker
  - Loop diuretic if fluid overload
  - Aldosterone antagonist (spironolactone)

- » If shock develops may support with IABP or Impella

Restrictive Cardiomyopathy

- » Rare disease of the myocardium
- » Restrictive filling of stiff ventricle(s) that don't relax
  - Can cause valvular regurgitation & back up to the atria & lungs
- » Ejection fraction & wall thickness is normal
- » Need fixed stroke volume
- » Over time may develop heart failure

Causes:

- » Amyloidosis (most common cause)
  - Abnormal protein build up
- » Hemochromatosis
  - Excessive iron
- » Sarcoidosis
- » Connective tissue disorders
- » Radiation and chemotherapy

Treatment:

- » Diuretics
  - Aldosterone antagonists (Spironolactone)
  - Heart failure meds with caution (hypotension)
- » Anti-arrhythmics
  - If issues with arrhythmias
- » Steroids (if indicated)
- » Chemotherapy for some causes

You Can Do It!

Chapter 5

Valvular Dysfunction, Inflammatory Diseases & Other Cardiac Issues

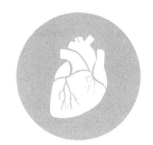

Topics covered in this chapter include:

- Murmurs & Valvular Dysfunction
- Valvular Disorders (stenosis & regurgitation)
  - Aortic, Mitral, Pulmonic & Tricuspid
- Acute Inflammatory Diseases
  - Myocarditis, Endocarditis & Pericarditis
- Cardiac tamponade
- Ventricular aneurysm

Murmurs & Valve Dysfunction

Murmurs—2 causes:

StenOsis:

» Forward flow of blood through stenotic open valves

Insufficiency/Regurgitation:

» Backward flow through incompetent closed valves

» Murmurs are high pitched except murmurs of stenosis

Systolic murmurs

» Pulmonic & aortic stenOsis are systolic murmurs...
- Murmurs of stenOsis are auscultated when valves are Open!
- The pulmonic & aortic valves are Open during systole
- Therefore, they are systolic murmurs!

» Tricuspid & mitral regurg/insufficiency are systolic murmurs...
- Murmurs of insufficiency are auscultated when valves are closed!
- The tricuspid & mitral valves are closed during systole
- Therefore, they are systolic murmurs!

» Auscultate on & between S_1 and S_2 (during systole)

» S_1 - murmur - S_2

Diastolic murmurs

» Tricuspid & mitral sten**O**sis are diastolic murmurs...
- Murmurs of sten**O**sis are auscultated when valves are **O**pen!
- The tricuspid & mitral valves are **O**pen during diastole
- Therefore, they are diastolic murmurs!

» Pulmonic & aortic regurgitation/insufficiency are diastolic murmurs...
- Murmurs of insufficiency are auscultated when valves are closed!
- The pulmonic & aortic & mitral valves are closed during diastole
- Therefore, they are diastolic murmurs

» Auscultate after S_2 (during diastole)

» S_1 - S_2 - murmur

Type of murmur	Systolic or Diastolic?	Location
Mitral Stenosis	Diastolic	5th ICS, MCL (M)
Mitral Regurg	Systolic	5th ICS, MCL (M)
Aortic Stenosis	Systolic	2nd ICS, RSB (A)
Aortic Regurg	Diastolic	2nd ICS, RSB (A)

Valvular Dysfunction

Mitral Insufficiency/Regurgitation

Causes:

» MI

» Ruptured chordae tendineae

» Severe left heart failure

» Left ventricular hypertrophy

» Hypertrophic Cardiomyopathy

» Mitral valve prolapse

» Rheumatic Heart Disease

» Myxomatous degeneration

» Endocarditis

Symptoms:

- » **SYSTOLIC murmur**
- » Orthopnea/dyspnea
- » Fatigue
- » Angina
- » Increased left atrial pressure
- » Right heart failure, over time can lead to left heart failure
- » Prone to atrial fibrillation d/t left atrial enlargement

Treatment:

- » Medical management targeted to reduce preload & afterload
- » Mitral valve clip (if a candidate)
  - Mitraclip®
- » Mitral valve replacement

Mitral Stenosis

- » Auscultate when the mitral valve is OPEN
- » Diastolic murmur

Signs & symptoms:

- » Pinkish cheeks
- » Pulmonary edema
- » Prone to afib
  - Due to atrial enlargement
- » ↑ right heart pressures
- » Pulmonary hypertension

Treatment:

- » **Medical management**
  - Aimed at reducing preload & afterload
- » Surgical replacement
- » Balloon Valvuloplasty
  - Increases the diameter of the valve
- » Valve repair/Commissurotomy

Mitral Valve Dysfunction:

Atrial enlargement is often seen with mitral valve dysfunction
This makes patients prone to atrial fibrillation
What you might see on the 12 Lead ECG:

» **Right atrial enlargement:**
- P wave amplitude > 2.5 mm in II &/or > 1.5 mm in V1
- QR, Qr, qR, or qRs morphology in lead V1 (without CAD)

» **Left atrial enlargement:**
- P wave duration ≥ 0.12 sec (usually lead II)
- Notched P wave in limb leads with the inter-peak duration ≥ 0.04 sec

» **Bi-atrial enlargement:**
- Features of both RAE and LAE in same ECG
- P wave in lead II > 2.5 mm tall and ≥ 0.12 sec in duration

Aortic Insufficiency/Regurgitation

Causes:

» Chronic hypertension

» Rheumatic Heart Disease

» Infective Endocarditis (IE)

» Marfan's Syndrome

» Idiopathic—means we don't know why!

» Acute AI-aortic dissection, endocarditis
- Go into shock
- Left ventricle can't handle excess volume

Physiologic changes:

» Results in a backflow of blood & reduced diastolic pressure

» Increased left ventricular volume

» **Hyperdynamic left ventricle**
- SV ↑ up to 3x normal to maintain CO

» **Over time, leads to left ventricular hypertrophy**
- Acute AI not tolerated well!

Signs & symptoms:

- » Diastolic murmur
- » Brisk carotid upstroke
- » DeMusset sign—head bobbing
- » Dyspnea/orthopnea
- » Warm & flushed
- » Wide pulse pressure - > 40 mm Hg
  - • High/normal systolic BP; low diastolic BP
- » "Water-hammer" pulse— rapid upstroke & down stroke with a shortened peak

Treatment:

- » Surgical valve replacement
- » IABP contraindicated!
- » Valve repair may be done as a palliative measure

Aortic Stenosis

- » Auscultate when the aortic valve is OPEN
- » Systolic murmur
- » Systolic ejection is impeded
- » Pressure gradient between LV & aorta
  - • Pressure higher in LV
- » 50%, 2-year mortality if HF develops

Symptoms:

- » Activity intolerance
- » SOB
- » Angina
- » Syncope
- » Chronic ↑ afterload due to narrow stenotic valve
  - • Leads to left ventricular hypertrophy
- » Heart failure
  - • Can develop reduced EF

Treatment:

- » Transcatheter Aortic Valve Replacement (TAVR)
- » Surgical valve replacement

Transcatheter Aortic Valve Replacement (TAVR)

- » Procedure for aortic stenosis
- » Replace aortic valve while heart is still beating
- » Post-procedure:
  - Monitor insertion site for bleeding, hematoma
  - Femoral access (most common)
  - Trans-carotid access
  - Trans-axillary access
- » Monitor for signs of stroke
  - Risk of plaque embolization
- » Bradycardia/Heart Block
  - May need permanent pacemaker long term
  - Incidence ~10%

Valvular diagnosis

- » Echocardiogram (gold standard)
- » Cardiac catheterization
  - May see ↓ CO, ↑ atrial pressure, ↑ PAOP, ↑ LVEDP
- » 12 lead ECG: left atrial & ventricular hypertrophy
- » Chest x-ray: left atrial & ventricular enlargement, pulmonary venous congestion

Treatment:

- » Treat heart failure if present:
  - ACE inhibitor, ARB or ARNI
    - ▷ Blunt RAAS
  - Beta blocker
    - ▷ Blunt the SNS
  - Diuretics
- Afterload reduction
  - ▷ Hydralazine, ACE Inhibitor or ARB
- » Valve repair/replacement

Acute Inflammatory Diseases

Myocarditis

- » Focal or diffuse inflammation of the myocardium
- » Viral or bacterial infection

Clinical signs:

- » Fever, chest pain, heart failure, dysrhythmias, sudden cardiac death
- » May be accompanied by pericarditis

Treatment:

- » Antibiotics (if bacterial)
- » NSAIDs
- » Diuretics

- » ACE inhibitor/ARBs
  - Goal is to ↓ afterload
  - Can also use vasodilators in the acute phase
- » + Inotropes
  - Improve contractility

Pericarditis

- » Inflammation of the pericardial sac
- » Constrictive: fibrous deposits on the pericardium
- » Restrictive: effusions into the pericardial sac

Causes:

- » Acute MI, post-CABG, connective tissue disease, infection
  - 10 - 15% develop this 2 - 7 days after AMI
- » Dressler's syndrome
  - 2 - 12 weeks after MI
  - Caused from an autoimmune response or viral infection

Valvular Dysfunction, Inflammatory Diseases & Other Cardiac Issues

Symptoms:

- » Retrosternal PLEURITIC chest pain
- » Pain is worse:
  - On inspiration (deep breath)
  - Supine position
  - With activity
- » Pain is relieved by leaning forward
- » Pericardial friction rub
- » Tachycardia
- » Tachyprea
- » Fever

Infective Endocarditis (IE)

- » Infection of the endocardium or valve
- » Damaged leaflets
- » Mitral valve most common in IE, then aortic, then combo mitral & aortic, then tricuspid; pulmonic is rare

Causes/at risk:

- » Prosthetic valves
- » Intra-cardiac devices (ICD, pacemaker)
- » Bacteria from other sources
- » IV drug abuse
- » At risk: cardiac surgery, rheumatic heart disease, dental procedures

Symptoms:

- » Stabbing, sharp pain
  - Worse on inspiration
  - May radiate to the neck, shoulders, back & arms
- » SOB, cough
- » JVD
- » Fever
- » Pulsus paradoxus
- » Pericardial friction rub
- » ST elevations on ECG
- » Narrow pulse pressure

- » Elevated WBC, ESR
- » Osler's nodes
  - Painful subcutaneous lesions in the fingers
- » Janeway lesions
  - Painless hemorrhagic lesions on the palms & soles

Complications of IE:

- » Heart failure
- » Valvular insufficiency
- » Renal failure
- » Stroke
- Vegetation embolism leading to stroke
- » 25% risk of death

Endocarditis common organisms:

- » Staphylococcus aureus – most common*
- » Streptococcus
- » Enterococcus
- » Gram negative bacilli
- » Fungus (i.e. candida)

Treatment:

- » Administer appropriate antibiotics
- » Usually high dose IV antibiotics
- » Surgical debridement with valve replacement

Various cardiac assessment findings with inflammatory diseases:

Pulsus paradoxus

- » Decrease in systolic pressure during inspiration
  - 10 mm Hg drop or more
- » Caused by cardiac tamponade, pleural effusion, pericarditis or dehydration

Pulsus alternans

» Finding on arterial waveform showing alternating strong & weak beats

» Indicative of left ventricular systolic impairment

Pericardial Rubs

» Scratching, grating, squeaking leather quality

» High frequency

» Left lower sternal border, leaning forward or lying supine in deep expiration

» 3 sounds are present
- One systolic – occurs anywhere in systole
- Two diastolic – occurs w/ ventricular stretch at early and late diastole

» Auscultated in MI, pericarditis, autoimmune, trauma, s/p cardiac surgery, autoimmune diseases

Overall "itis" treatment goals:

» Prevent/relieve symptoms (lean forward)

» NSAIDs
- Ibuprofen
- Indomethacin
- Colchicine

» Treat infection

» Corticosteroids

» Chronic: partial pericardiectomy
- Window is created allowing fluids to drain into pleural space

» Constrictive pericarditis: total pericardiectomy

Cardiac Tamponade

- » Compression of the heart due to blood or fluid accumulation within the pericardium

- » The pericardial space normally contains 20 – 50 ml of pericardial fluid

- » Clinical signs/symptoms of cardiac tamponade:
  - **Beck's Triad**:
    - ▷ Elevated CVP w/JVD
    - ▷ Hypotension
    - ▷ Muffled heart sounds
  - CVP & PAOP "Rise & equalize"

- » Wide mediastinum on chest xray

- » Sudden drop in chest tube output

- » Narrow pulse pressure (SBP – DBP = PP)
  - Normal PP = 40 mm Hg

- » Tachycardia

- » Electrical alternans
  - Alternating beat variation of amplitude on ECG

- » Pulsus paradoxus
  - > 10 mm Hg drop in BP during inspiration

- » Cardiac Arrest
  - Vfib/PEA

Treatment of cardiac tamponade:

- » Pericardiocentesis if absence of myocardial compression
  - Pericardial effusion

- » Sternotomy in emergency
  - Resternotomy post CABG to locate & control source of bleeding
  - Myocardial compression

Ventricular Aneurysm

- » Bulge or 'pocketing' of the wall or lining of a vessel in the left ventricle
  - Swells into a "bubble" of blood
  - Can form in the blood vessels at the base of the septum, or within the aorta
- » Can happen after a myocardial infarction – usually develop slowly

Symptoms:

- » May see ST elevation on 12 Lead ECG
- » Depending on the size, it may impede blood flow to the body
- » Clots can form within the aneurysm
- » Monitor for signs of embolism:
  - CVA symptoms
  - Limb ischemia

Diagnosis:

- » ECHO

Treatment:

- » They may not need treatment
- » Anticoagulation to prevent thrombus formation
- » ACE Inhibitors may be preventative after MI
- » Surgery – ventricular reduction

You Can Do It!

Chapter 6
Arrhythmias & Cardiac Arrest

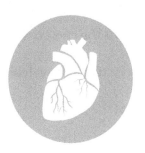

Topics covered in this chapter include:

- Tachydysrhythmias
- Bradydysrhythmias
- Conduction defects & blocks – See Acute Coronary Syndrome section
- Emergent transcutaneous & transvenous pacing
- Genetic Cardiac Disease
  - Long QT Syndrome (LQTS)
  - Brugada Syndrome
- Cardiac Arrest & Resuscitation
- Post arrest care
- Targeted Temperature Management (TTM)

Atrial Fibrillation (A. Fib)

Known as the "neuro rhythm" because of the embolic stroke incidence

Risk factors for developing Afib/aflutter:

- CABG
- Valvular disease
- MI/atherosclerosis
- Atrial enlargement
- Heart failure
- Rheumatic Heart Disease
- Lung Disease
- Obesity

Rates can vary: > 100 "Rapid ventricular response"

- Lose atrial kick
- ↓ in C.O. by up to 20 - 25%

Management:

- You need to decide to rate control vs. rhythm conversion or both
- In chronic afib, would never want to convert unless you confirm via TEE no thrombus present
- In chronic afib, thrombi most often form in the left atrium & left atrial appendage
- Anticoagulation is necessary

Atrial Fibrillation management:

- Emergent synchronized cardioversion if new (vs. chronic) & UNSTABLE!!
- With antidysrhythmic use, it is key to know the patient's EF/heart function
- Amiodarone – safer to use with reduced ejection fraction
- Beta blockers* (Ex. Esmolol, metoprolol)
- Calcium channel blockers* (Ex. diltiazem)
  - *Use cautiously in patients with reduced EF
- Digoxin
- Anticoagulation if sustained afib

Medications:

Amiodarone

- » Used to treat atrial or ventricular arrhythmias
- » Effects mostly K⁺ channels in myocardial cells
- » Atrial arrhythmias – dose 150 mg over 10 min IV, then 1 mg/min x 6 hours, then 0.5 mg/min x 18 hours
  - Transition to PO dosing after IV is complete if needed
- » Adverse effects - Monitor QTc interval, as it will prolong
- » Hypotension, bradycardia
- » Long term use: toxicity, pulmonary fibrosis, neuro or hepatic injury, thyroid dysfunction
- » Has a loooooooooooong half-life of about 58 days!!!! Whoa!

Beta Blockers

Metoprolol (Lopressor)

- » Selectively blocks beta$_1$ receptors
- » Effects: reduces HR, prolongs AV node conduction, suppresses renin secretion
- » Negative inotrope, so decreases contractility & C.O.
  - Decreases workload of heart (long term)
- » Dose: 5 mg every 5 min up to about 15 mg
- » Adverse effects: bradycardia, hypotension, heart failure, hypoglycemia
- » Use with caution in asthmatic patients!

Esmolol (Brevibloc)

- » Selectively blocks beta$_1$ receptors
- » Used to treat SVT, rate control for A. Fib & flutter, HTN

» Dose: Bolus 500 mcg/kg/min (over 1 min), then start infusion at 50 mcg/kg/min & increase by 50 mcg/kg/min every 5 – 10 min

» Maximum is about 200 mcg/kg/min infusion

» Short half-life, so if patient develops side effects, shut it off

» Adverse effects: hypotension, bradycardia, heart block, heart failure, bronchospasm

Calcium Channel Blockers

Diltiazem (Cardizem)

» Negative chronotropic effects (potent) & mild negative inotropic effects

» Used in A. Fib, A. flutter & PSVT

» Also used to treat angina, HTN

» Dose: Push 5 – 20 mg IV, then start infusion 5 – 15 mg/hr

» Adverse effects: Hypotension, 2nd or 3rd degree AV block, bradycardia, asystole, heart failure, N/V

Other options

Digoxin/Lanoxin

» **Loading dose: 1.0 - 1.5 mg over 24 hours**
  - Average dose is 0.125 - 0.25 mg daily

» **Therapeutic range 0.5 - 2.0 ng/mL**
  - Check level 6 - 8 hours after dose

» **Digoxin can cause almost any arrhythmia**

» **Digoxin effects & uses:**
  - Increases myocardial contractility
  - Slows conduction of impulse through the AV node
  - Used to control ventricular rate in atrial fibrillation or atrial flutter
    ▷ May be best suited for use in patients with heart failure & atrial fibrillation

» **In heart failure—does not reduce mortality, but may be helpful for symptom control**

» **Know apical HR & K+ before giving**

- Hypokalemia ↑ risk of Digoxin toxicity

» **Consider renal function (note creatinine level)**

» **Signs of Digoxin toxicity:**
  - Bradycardia
  - Prolonged PR interval – 1st degree AV conduction delay
  - ST segmented depression
  - Prolonged QT interval
  - Vision changes, see yellow halos
  - Nausea/vomiting
  - Dizziness

» **Digoxin toxicity reversal: Digibind (digoxin immune fab)**
  - Binds to Dig in the extracellular space
  - Start to see improvement ~30 min.

» **Look for meds that increase or decrease the effects of digoxin:**
  - Amiodarone
    ▷ Increases Dig levels
    ▷ Decrease dose by 1/2 when amiodarone is started
  - PPIs
    ▷ Increases Dig levels
  - Antacids
    ▷ Decreases bioavailability of Dig

MAZE Procedure

» **Long term treatment of atrial fibrillation**

» **Surgical incisions made in the left & right atrium in a maze pattern to form scar tissue**

» **Scar tissue doesn't conduct erratic impulses**

» **Redirects the electrical impulse**

Atrial flutter

» **Atrial rates 240 – 400 beats/min, ventricular rates can vary**
  - Ventricular rates can be faster than afib & more difficult to control
  - ↓ CO from RVR

» **AV node conduction block**

» **Symptoms: Syncope, palpitations, fatigue, exercise intolerance, SOB, chest pain**

» **~ 60% have underlying CAD**
  - Sequelae of open heart surgery

- » Catheter ablation is superior (long term) to rate & rhythm control
  - TTE – preferred method for evaluating atrial flutter
  - TEE – best for viewing left atrium for thrombus
- » Short term - High success with cardioversion
- » Risk: Thrombus formation
  - Anticoagulate > 48 hours or uncertain onset

Supraventricular Tachycardia (SVT)

Always ask:

- » Stable vs. unstable?
- » Unstable: prepare for synchronized cardioversion!
- » Stable: remember VAD!

If stable, remember this acronym: VAD

- » **V**agal maneuvers
- » **A**denosine 6 mg IV - Rapid!!!
  - Repeat 12 mg x 2, every 1 - 2 min
- » **D**iltiazem IV or beta blocker

Adenosine administration

- » Depresses AV node conduction & SA node activity, used in SVT
- » Half-life is seconds! < 10 seconds
- » Dosed: 6 mg, 12 mg & repeat 12 mg RAPID IVP over 1 - 2 seconds, follow by flush
  - Use IV closest to the heart
- » Instruct patient prior to administration, patient may feel breathless or have transient chest pain
- » Adverse effects: transient asystole or AV block, facial flushing, hypotension, nausea (all brief)
- » DO NOT use in heart blocks, WPW with wide QRS, asthma/bronchospasm

Tachycardia – Wide complex

- » QRS > 0.12 sec: consult an expert
- » Leads V1 & V6 best for differentiating SVT vs. ventricular origin
- » Monitor electrolytes
  - K^+, Mg^{++}, Ca^{++}
- » Amiodarone 150 mg IV over 10 min
- » Can also use Lidocaine for monomorphic wide complex tachycardia
- » Since 2010 guidelines:
  - Adenosine 6 mg IV, may repeat dose

Wolfe-Parkinson-White (WPW)

- » Pre-excitation
- » Abnormal conduction pathway between the atria & ventricles
  - Often use Bundle of Kent accessory pathway
- » Accessory pathways conduct faster than the AV node
- » Short PR interval < 0.12 sec
- » Delta wave—slurred upstroke in the QRS

Treatment:

- » Antiarrhythmic medications slow conduction
  - Beta blockers often used
  - Other options: flecainide, propafenone, sotalol, or amiodarone
- » Avoid digoxin, calcium channel blockers & adenosine
- » Can cardiovert in the short term if unstable
- » Long term: EP consult for ablation of the accessory pathway

Antidysrhythmic Medications

» Monitor leads V1 &/or V6

» Monitor QTc interval with administration of antidysthythmic medications

Antidysrhythmic Medications:

Class	Medication	Effect	Uses
IA	Quinidine (Cardioquin)* Procainamide (Pronestyl)*	Prolongs repolarization	Atrial or ventricular dysrhythmia monitor QTc interval - will prolong
IB	Lidocaine (Xylocaine)* Tocainamide (Tonocard) Mexiletin (Mexitil)	Shortens action potential duration	Ventricular dysrhythmias
IC	Flecainamide (Tambocor) Propafenone (Rhythmol)	Blocks Na+ channels	Ventricular dysrhythmias
II	Propanolol (Inderal) Esmolol (Brevibloc)*	Decreases HR & SA node automaticity Beta blocker	Atrial dysrhythmias & SVT
III	Amiodarone (Cordarone)** Bretylium (Bretylol) Sotalol (Betapace)	Blocks K+ channels, slows conduction	Atrial & ventricular dysrhythmias
IV	Verapamil (Calan)* Diltiazem (Cardizem)*	Calcium channel antagonist	Atrial tachycardia & atrial flutter
Other	Digoxin (Lanoxin)* Adenosine (Adenocard)*	Slows AV node conduction, depresses SA node	Atrial fibrilation, atrial flutter & SVT

Pacemaker Review

» Permanent or temporary

» Indications:
- Symptomatic bradycardia
- 2nd Degree AV Block (Mobitz II)
- Third Degree AV Block

» Patients admitted with "Syncope" will require f/u EP study

» Transcutaneous, transvenous, epicardial
- Options to emergently pace

NBG 3 letter pacing codes:

First: Chamber paced	Second: Chamber sensed	Third: Response to sensing
A = Atrium	A = Atrium	I = Inhibited
V = Ventricle	V = Ventricle	(if QRS is sensed)
D = Dual (A & V)	D = Dual (A & V)	T = Triggered
O = None	O = None	D = Inhibited & triggered
		O = None
TCP & TVP only uses "V"	TCP & TVP only uses "V"	"I" is preferred This is Demand pacing!

Example: VVI mode – V: ventricle is paced, V: ventricle is sensed, I: pacing inhibited if the pacemaker senses intrinsic conduction

Pacing Modes

» **Modes: Synchronous (demand) or Asynchronous (non-demand)**
  - In almost all instances, you want to be in Synchronous (demand) mode
  - It will only pace when the patient needs it (i.e. heart rate falls below the set pacemaker rate)
  - Synchronous mode avoids a pacing stimulus delivered during repolarization...this is bad because it could cause R on T and ventricular dysrhythmias & death

**Asynchronous is dangerous if the patient has any underlying rhythm!!!!
  - In general, avoid asynchronous mode!

» **Emergent temporary pacing: demand mode should be used**

» **Transcutaneous or transvenous**
  - Epicardial pacing is used in cardiac surgery - not tested on this exam!

Transcutaneous Pacing (TCP)

» **External stimulation of the heart through pacing pads**

» **Pad placement: anterior – posterior or anterior – lateral**

Settings:

- **Mode: Demand (synchronous) – the only mode is VVI**
  - Fixed (asynchronous) – again, AVOID!

- **In general, start @ 50 mA Energy:**
  - Increase the mA (energy) until you see a pacing spike immediately followed by a wide QRS complex
  - Set the mA above where capture was achieved (gives a safety margin)
  - Need higher energy because stimulus needs to pace through skin, bone & muscle
  - The wide QRS is normal because one side of the heart is being stimulated & the impulse waves across the myocardium to depolarize

- **Rate: There's no magic to this, if the BP is in the toilet, increase the rate!**
  - Remember, cardiac output = HR x SV
  - What can you manipulate? HR!
  - Palpate pulse
  - Assess BP to verify effective capture (BP should improve)

Other important concepts:

- **More energy required with TCP vs. transvenous (start @ 50 mA & increase until capture)**
  - Once capture is achieved, add an extra 10 mA to give the patient a safety margin
  - Energy requirements will vary from patient to patient

- **Not as effective as transvenous & should only be used until you can TVP!**

- **Consider pain medication/ sedation, as TCP is uncomfortable!**

- **Prepare for TVP insertion!**

Transvenous Pacing (TVP)

- » Pacing wire is inserted into the right ventricle through an introducer
- » Can only pace the right ventricle (VVI)
- » Most wires are bipolar
  - Both poles are in the heart
  - The (-) pole is in contact with the myocardium
  - Returns to the (+) pole
  - Very small or absent pacing spike
- » Less energy required vs. TCP

Initial settings:

- » Set the **pacing mode**
  - You want to be in demand mode, so the pacer can see or sense the patient's intrinsic rhythm
- » Set the **pacing rate**
  - ~ 60 - 80 bpm or whatever the patient needs!
- » Set the **pacing output (energy)**
  - Measured in milliamps (mA)
  - ~ 5 mA
- » Set the **pacing sensitivity**
  - Measured in millivolts (mV)
  - ~2 mV
- » Assess for capture – electrical (+/- pacing spike & wide QRS) & mechanical (pulse palpated)
- » Secure wires

Issues with Pacing:

Failure to capture

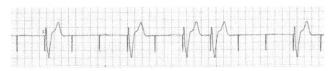

Electrical stimulus delivered (pacing spike), but no electrical capture (wide QRS)

Chapter 6

Causes:

- » Improper position of wire or pads
- » Low voltage (mA)
  - Increase the mA setting!
- » Battery failure
- » Inadequate connection
- » Fibrosis of catheter tip
  - Transvenous wire
- » Acidosis or hypoxia – may need higher energy setting

Trouble-shooting:

- » Check connections
- » Increase mA (energy)
- » Assess pH, electrolyte imbalances, ischemia & drug toxicity
  - May require much higher mA to capture

Failure to pace

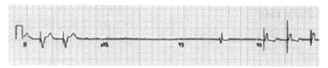

A pacing stimulus is not delivered

Causes:

- » Battery failure
- » Pad or lead dislodgement
- » Generator failure
- » Improper settings
- » Sensitivity (mV) setting is too low

Troubleshooting:

- » Assess leads & connections
- » Assess labs
- » Assess sensitivity threshold
- » Change battery
- » Change the generator
- » Prepare for TCP

Failure to sense:

- » **Under-sensing:** the pacemaker does not recognize intrinsic beats
  - Dangerous, because patient can experience R on T phenomenon

- » **Over-sensing:** the pacemaker thinks that either p waves or t waves are ventricular depolarization & may not deliver a pacing stimulus

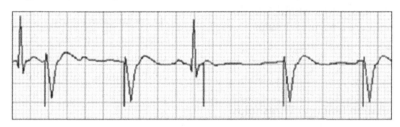

This is an example of under-sensing. The pacemaker didn't "see" or sense the R wave & a pacing spike is seen on the the T wave.

Causes:

- » *Improper sensitivity settings
- » **Position of the lead**
- » **Rhythm strip above is an example of under-sensing**
  - This can lead to R on T arrhythmia - dangerous!
  - Pacing spikes where they shouldn't be
  - Sensitivity setting (mV) is too high (least sensitive or asynchronous mode)
  - Action: decrease sensitivity setting/number (mV), making the pacemaker more sensitive!

- » **Can also be a sensitivity issue when pacing spikes aren't delivered when they should be**
  - Sensitivity setting (mV) is too low (most sensitive)
  - Most sensitive setting – pacer senses P &/or T waves & thinks it is ventricular depolarization
  - Action: increase sensitivity setting/number (mV), making the pacemaker less sensitive!

Troubleshooting:

» Assess thresholds

Assessing Pacemaker Thresholds:

» **Stimulation (energy) threshold**
  - *Goal:* to use the least amount of energy as possible, but still capture a pacing stimulus

» **Sensing threshold**
  - *Goal:* prevent competitive pacing

» **Thresholds are only assessed if the patient has an underlying rhythm & is hemodynamically stable!**

Stimulation (energy) Threshold:

» **Increase pacing rate on the generator above patient's intrinsic rate**

» **Increase output (mA) to obtain 1:1 capture**

» **While watching the monitor, decrease the output (mA)**
  - Note when there is no longer capture

» **Increase mA until 1:1 capture resumes**
  - This is the pacing threshold
  - Set mA 2 – 3 x's above threshold

» **Return rate to previous rate setting**

Sensitivity Threshold:

» **Decrease the mA to lowest setting (0.1 mA)**

» **Turn the pacing rate to 10 beats below the patient's intrinsic rate**

» **While watching the sense light on the pacemaker, slowly increase the sensitivity value (mV) - making it <u>less</u> sensitive (bigger mV value)**

» **Watch for the flashing indicator lights**
  - Green: pacing, orange: sensing

» **Note when the <u>sensitivity</u> indicator stops flashing with each QRS**
  - This is the sensitivity threshold
  - Set the sensitivity at ½ the threshold

Least sensitive:
mV set at 20 or asynchronous...
doesn't see the R wave

This is where you want the sensitivity to be...the pacemaker can sense or "see" the QRS, but not the P & the T

Most sensitive
mV set at 0.5 ...may see P's and T's & think it's an R wave, a pacing stimulus is not delivered

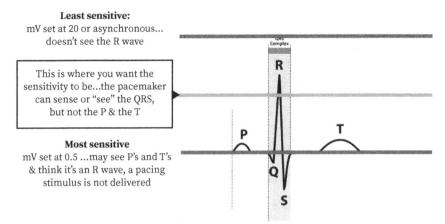

Sensitivity issues:

Under-sensing:

» Pacing spikes where they shouldn't be!

» The pacemaker does not recognize intrinsic beats

- R on T & can cause arrhythmias

» Treatment: DEcrease the mV value making it MORE sensitive

» Too sensitive

Over-sensing:

- May not pace when it needs to
- Don't see pacing spikes (or paced rhythm) when you should
- The pacemaker sees P or T waves & thinks it doesn't need to pace

» Treatment: INcrease the mV value making it LESS sensitive

Nursing care of transvenous paced patients:

» Immobilize affected extremity

» Monitor pulses distal to insertion site

» Bedrest especially if patient is pacer dependent!

» Daily chest x-ray to assess wire placement

» Do not bolus fluids through the introducer (can dislodge the wire)

Other tips:

- » Assess thresholds daily if hemodynamically stable
- » Monitor for signs of perforation!
  - Hiccups are a sign of perforation – stimulating or pacing the diaphragm
  - Watch for signs of tamponade

Magnet Operation with Permanent Pacemakers & ICDs

- » A magnet placed over a pacemaker causes asynchronous pacing at a designated "magnet" rate
  - Does NOT turn off the pacemaker...a common misconception!!!
- » Over an ICD, a magnet inhibits defibrillation
- » A magnet might be used in surgery if cautery is used or if a defibrillator is mis-firing
- » Terminates pacemaker mediated tachycardia

Genetic Cardiac Disease

Long QT syndrome (LQTS)

- » Delayed repolarization can cause Torsade de Pointes
  - Polymorphic ventricular tachycardia
- » Present with fainting or sudden cardiac death
- » Prolonged QT, QTc > 450 ms
- » Can also result from malnutrition due to K^+ & Mg^+ deficiencies

Treatment:

- » Genetic testing
- » Electrolyte supplements
- » Beta blockers
- » Antidysrhythmic based on cause of LQTS
- » Implantable cardioverter defibrillator (ICD)

Brugada Syndrome

- » Genetic cause of sudden cardiac death
- » Sodium channelopathy

Symptoms:

- » Fainting, irregular heart beats
- » Coved or saddle-back ST elevations in leads V1 – V3
- » Often have a right BBB
- » Long PR interval
- » May have short QT interval; < 360 ms
- » Structural right ventricle pathology

Treatment:

- » Implantable cardioverter defibrillator (ICD)
- » Possibly quinidine

Cardiac Arrest & Resuscitation

- » **Early CPR with minimal interruptions**
- » **Compressions of good quality**
  - 100 - 120/minute
  - 2 - 2.4 inch depth
- » **Early defibrillation**
  - Minimize pauses
  - Escalate energy
- » **Avoid excessive ventilation**
  - 10 breaths/min or 30:2
- » **Figure out cause**
  - 5 H's, 5 T's

Types of arrest & treatment strategies:

Ventricular Fibrillation

- **S**hock (if readily available); Repeat Q 2 min.
- **C**PR for 2 min, minimize pauses!
- **R**hythm check - shock if warranted
- **E**pi 1 mg IV/IO Q 3 - 5 min
- **A**miodarone 300 mg IV/IO; repeat bolus 150 mg IV/IO if still in VF/VT
- **M**edications (other): Lidocaine 1.0 - 1.5 mg/kg IV/IO

Torsades de pointes

- "Polymorphic" ventricular tachycardia
- Shift in axis
- Caused by hypomagnesemia, prolonged QT, multiple medications
- Also caused by methadone & some quinolones
  - ▷ Causes prolonged QT interval
- Treatment: magnesium sulfate 1 - 2 grams IV/IO (diluted)
- Magnesium antagonist: calcium chloride

PEA (pulseless electrical activity)

- **P**ump: Start compressions
- **E**pinephrine 1 mg IV/IO Q 3 - 5 min
- **A**ssess causes

Asystole

- No cardiac output
- **P**ump (Same as PEA)
- **E**pinephrine 1 mg IV/IO Q 3 - 5 min
- **A**ssess causes
- Consider termination if Capnography < 10 mm Hg after 20 min

Figure out the cause: 5 H's & 5 T's

» **5 H's:**
- Hypovolemia
- Hypoxia
- Hypo/Hyperkalemia
- H+ ion (acidosis)
- Hypothermia

» **5 T's:**
- Thrombus:
  ▷ MI
  ▷ PE
- Tension pneumothorax
- Tamponade
- Toxicology (drug OD)

Capnography during resuscitation

» **Normal PEtCO$_2$ 35 - 45 mm Hg**

» **Minimum goal > 10 mm Hg**

» **Used as a marker of perfusion & chest compression quality**

» **If < 10, improve quality of compressions**

» **If rapid increase in PEtCO$_2$, may be a sign of ROSC**

» **If consistently < 10 mm Hg in the setting of adequate compressions, discuss termination of resuscitation efforts**
- Unless it is a suspected pulmonary embolism

Post-arrest care

» Optimize hemodynamics
- Avoid hypotension
- Avoid hypoxemia or hyperoxemia

» Reperfusion
- Obtain 12 Lead ECG
- Does the patient need to go to the Cath lab?

» Targeted Temperature Management (TTM)

Targeted Temperature Management (TTM)

Previously referred to as "Therapeutic Hypothermia"

Treatment: Target 32°C – 36°C for 24 hours post arrest

» Select a temperature & stay there, don't let the patient vacillate

» Minimize reperfusion injury that leads to neuro damage

Cellular damage after cardiac arrest:

» O_2 & glucose stores depleted

» Intracellular calcium influx

» Formation of O_2 free radicals

» Release of glutamate

» Intracellular acidosis

» Disruption in blood brain barrier

» Mitochondrial injury

» Apoptosis

PEARLS:

- » 32°C – 36°C for 24 hours
- » Only in patients remaining comatose post cardiac arrest
- » AHA class I recommendation for all rhythms
  - Randomized controlled trials to support TTM
- » Neuro-protective
- » Avoid fever post TTM for at least 48 hours
- » Rewarm slowly to a normal temperature

Side effects of cooling:

- » Shivering
  - Aggressively treat it!
- » Bradycardia (seen more with 32°C – 34 °C range)
  - Only treat if hypotensive
- » Vasoconstriction induced hypertension
- » Diuresis (seen more with 32°C – 34 °C range)
- » Hypokalemia/ electrolyte shifting (seen more with 32°C – 34 °C range)
- » Elevated lactate
  - Clears when the patient rewarms

You Can Do It!

Chapter 7
Vascular issues

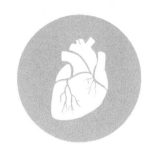

Topics covered in this chapter include:

- Hypertension & Hypertensive emergencies
- Aortic aneurysm – abdominal & thoracic
- Acute arterial occlusion
- Acute venous thrombosis

Hypertension

Category	SBP		DBP
Normal	< 120	and	< 80
Elevated	120 - 129	and	< 80
Stage 1 HTN	130 - 139	or	80-89
Stage 2 HTN	≥ 140	or	≥ 90
Hypertensive urgency	> 180	and/or	> 120

Source: AHA Hypertension Guidelines

Long term BP Goals:

» < 130/80

First line medications recommended for general hypertension management:

» **Thiazide diuretic**
  - Longer acting preferred

» **Calcium channel blocker**
  - "dipines"

» **ACE inhibitor**
  - "prils"

» **Angiotensin receptor blocker (ARB)**
  - "sartans"

Hypertensive Emergency

» SBP > 180 &/or DBP > 120

Acute BP elevation associated with organ damage

» Kidney: decreased blood flow, hematuria, proteinuria

» Brain: hypertensive encephalopathy

» Heart: LVH, LVF, MI

» Eyes: retinal hemorrhages

» Vascular system: vessel damage

Treatment:

- » BP in both arms
  - R/o aneurysm or steal syndrome
- » Decrease BP by 25% within 1 hour
- » IV anti-hypertensives (vasodilators, diuretics, etc.)
  - Beta blockers
    - ▷ Esmolol (Brevibloc)
    - ▷ Labetolol (Trandate)
    - ▷ Metoprolol (Lopressor)
- Nitrates
  - ▷ Nipride (Nitroprusside)
- Calcium channel blockers
  - ▷ Nicardipine (Cardene)
  - ▷ Clevidipine (Cleviplex)
- Hydralazine
- Fenoldopam (Corlopam)
- » Consider 12 Lead ECG

Aneurysms

Definition: permanent localized dilation of aorta 1.5 times diameter

- » Patients will describe "ripping" chest pain radiating to the back
- » > 6 cm associated with increased risk of rupture

Types:

- » Thoracic (TAA)
- » Abdominal (AAA)
- » Aortic dissection
- » Rupture – 90% mortality

Thoracic Aortic Aneurysm (TAA)

- » At risk: HTN, smoking
- » Dilatation of the aorta > 50% of its normal diameter
- » Goal: Prevent rupture or dissection

Treatment:

- » BP control/HR reduction
  - Beta blockers are key!
  - Reduce HR, BP & force of contraction
- » Surgical repair

Aortic Dissection

- » Hypertension is a major risk factor
- » Tear in the inner layer of the aorta

Symptoms:

- » BP difference of ≥ 25 mmHG between arms
- » Sudden, severe pain
- » Ripping or tearing pain radiating to back & neck
- » Shortness of breath
- » Muffled heart sounds
- » Tachycardia

Ascending TAA (Type A)

- » Life threatening
- » At risk for aortic insufficiency
- » Diastolic murmur
- » Widened pulse pressure
- » Bounding pulse

Treatment:

- » Emergent surgical repair or replace the proximal segment of the ascending aorta, +/- arch &/or valve

Descending aorta or aortic arch (Type B)

- » Descending tear
- » Can extend to the abdominal aorta

- » Intermittent or constant chest pain radiating to back
  - Dull pain between shoulders

Treatment:

- » Stat CT scan
- » Consider TEE
- » If dissected, administer vasodilators to keep BP controlled

- » Endovascular stenting
- » Surgical repair considered if > 6 cm in diameter
- » +/- Surgery depending on location and organs affected

Abdominal Aneurysm

- » Pulsation in the abdomen
- » Control HTN

- » Surgical repair

Signs of rupture:

- » Unrelenting back pain
- » Hypotension
- » Tachycardia

- » Shock
- » Carries ~90% mortality

Endovascular repair of aneurysms:

- » TEVAR: Thoracic endovascular aortic repair
- » Surgical repair concern: Aorta cross-clamping can lead to spinal cord ischemia/infarction

- » Paraplegia incidence:
  - Surgical TAAA incidence 8 – 28%
  - TEVAR incidence 4 – 7%

Blood Pressure Control

Beta Blockers

Esmolol (Brevibloc)

- » Short acting beta blocker
- » Initial dose:
  - 250 - 500 mcg/kg IV over 1 min
- » Maintenance dose:
  - 50 – 200 mcg/kg/min IV infusion

Labetalol (Trandate)

- » Blocks alpha, B_1 & B_2

Dosing:

- » 20 mg IV over 2 min
- » Follow with 20 - 80 mg IV q 10 - 15 min until BP is controlled
- » Maintenance dose:
  - 1-2 mg/min IV continuous infusion
  - Titrate up to 5 - 20 mg/min; not to exceed total dose of 300 mg

Metoprolol (Lopressor)

- » Dose: 5 mg IV q 2 min, up to 3 times

Other Vasodilators

Nitroprusside (Nipride)

- » Arterial & venous vasodilation

Dosing:

- » Starting dose: 0.3 mcg/kg/min
- » Maximum dose usually 10 mcg/kg/min

- » Monitor thiocyanate level for toxicity!
- • Toxicity develops with higher doses when used > 48 – 72°

Nicardipine (Cardene)

- » Calcium channel blocker
- » Direct arterial vasodilator
- » Dose: 5 – 15 mg/hr

Peripheral Arterial Disease

Lower extremity PAD

- » 60% have CAD
- » Atherosclerosis
- » Most common cause of death after vascular surgery is a MI
- » Claudication – can be intermittent with exercise
- » Limb ischemia

Risk factors:

- » Smoking
- » DM
- » Dyslipidemia
- » HTN
- » Age > 70

7 P's:

- » Pain
- » Pallor
- » Paresthesia
- » Paralysis
- » Pulseless
- » Poor temperature (polar)
- » Poor healing

Ankle/Brachial Index (ABI)

- » Arm pressure - SBP from brachial artery
- » Ankle pressure - SBP from posterior tibial & dorsalis pedis arteries
- » Divide ankle pressure by arm
- » ABI value > 0.9 normal
- » < 0.4 severe obstruction

Diagnostics/Treatment

- » Doppler studies
- » Arteriography

Management:

Goal is to improve perfusion!

- » Anticoagulation
  - Antiplatelet agents
  - Thrombolytic agents
- » Vasodilators
- » Angioplasty
- » Stents
- » Surgery – bypass
- » Amputation

Deep Venous Thrombosis (DVT)

- » Now called VTE – venous thromboembolism
- » May have pain &/or swelling in affected extremity
- » + Homans' sign
  - Pain in calf with abrupt dorsiflexion of the foot while the knee is flexed at 90°
  - Not a diagnostic indicator
- » If shortness of breath develops, consider pulmonary embolism
- » Anticoagulation usually with heparin short term, Coumadin long term
  - Direct oral anticoagulants (DOACs) are often used
- » **Consider IVC filter if lower extremity DVT**

Chapter 8
Other Patient Care Problems

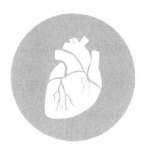

Topics covered in this chapter include:

- Hematology
  - Thrombocytopenia
  - Anticoagulation
  - Heparin Induced Thrombocytopenia (HIT)
- Neurology
  - Stroke
  - Carotid Stenosis
- Renal
  - Acute Kidney Injury
  - Contrast Induced Nephropathy
  - Dialysis (Hemodialysis & CRRT)
  - Air Embolism
  - Potassium, Magnesium & Calcium Imbalances
- Pulmonary
  - ABGs
  - Capnography
  - Non-Invasive Ventilation
  - ARDS
  - Pulmonary Embolism (PE)
  - Pulmonary Arterial Hypertension (PAH)

Hematology

Thrombocytopenia

- » Platelet count < 150,000 /uL

- » The body can form platelet plugs until the platelet count is about 100,000 /uL

- » Without a structural lesion, we can tolerate platelet count ~ 5,000 /uL as long as there is no major bleeding!

- » In ICUs, the incidence of thrombocytopenia is up to 35%

- » Causes of thrombocytopenia:
  - Sepsis - Phagocytosis of platelets by macrophages
  - DIC
  - Inflammation

Many medications cause impaired platelet function.

Here's a short list:

- » ASA
- » Clopidogrel
- » Prasugrel
- » Pradaxa
- » Glycoprotein inhibitors
- » Ticlidopine
- » Alteplase
- » Heparin
- » Dextran

- » Penicillin
- » Cephalosporin
- » Diphenhydramine
- » Calcium Channel Blockers
- » Nitroglycerin
- » Nitroprusside
- » Haloperidol
- » Ketorolac

Platelets

- Normal 150,000 – 400,000/uL
- Also called thrombocytes d/t their role in clotting
- ~65% of platelets circulate in blood, ~35% stored in spleen

Coagulopathies & Platelet Disorders

In thrombocytopenia, either:

- Not enough platelets or there is impaired function of the platelet
- Life span of a platelet is 10 days
- Any endothelial damage causes platelets to adhere to collagen

Clot formation:

1. Release of calcium
2. Activation of Glycoprotein IIb/IIIa receptors on the surface of platelets
3. GP IIb/IIIa receptors bind to fibrinogen to form bridges to other platelets to form clots
4. Calcium activates the coagulation cascade
5. End result → thrombus

Platelet Transfusions

- When whole blood is donated, platelets get separated with leukocytes
  - Increased incidence of fever with a platelet transfusion d/t leukocytes
- Banked platelets are usually pooled
- Store banked platelets up to 7 days
- Viability decreases after 3 days
- Pooled platelet transfusion
  - Should see a 30,000/uL rise
  - See increase 1 hour after transfusion, lasts 8 days

If not seeing an increase in the platelet count with a transfusion consider:

» Leukocyte reduced transfusion

» ABO compatibility

Heparin Induced Thrombocytopenia (HIT)

» Platelet count drops by ≥ 30 – 50% from baseline within 5 – 10 days of exposure to Heparin

» May develop more quickly if previous exposure to Heparin

» 25% of patients develop systemic reaction

- Fever
- Chills
- Tachypnea
- Tachycardia

» Erythematous lesions around SQ Heparin injection sites

» **Major complication: Thrombosis!

- DVT of lower extremity
- DVT of upper extremity
- Pulmonary embolus
- Arterial thrombosis
- AMI & stroke

» Risk is greater with unfractionated Heparin (UFH)

» Even low doses & heparin flushes!!!

» Don't forget: Heparin coated catheters!!!

Diagnosis of HIT:

» Clinical exposure to Heparin

» Thrombocytopenia

» Symptomatic thrombosis

» IgG Antibodies to Heparin

- Platelet Factor 4 complex
- IgG with Reflex to Serotonin Release Assay

» Clinical picture + assay for diagnosis

Treatment of HIT:

- » Discontinue all forms of Heparin!!!
- » Anticoagulation using Direct Thrombin Inhibitors (DTIs):
  - Bivalirudin (Angiomax)
    - ▷ Initial: 0.15 - 0.2 mg/kg/hr IV
    - ▷ Adjust to aPTT 1.5 - 2.5 times baseline value
    - ▷ Renal adjustments are necessary
  - Argatroban (Acova)
    - ▷ 2 mcg/kg/min - Max 10 mcg/kg/min
    - ▷ PTT 1.5 - 3 x baseline value, not to exceed 100 seconds
    - ▷ Cleared by the liver

- » Long term anticoagulation with Coumadin
- » Heparin antibodies may last > 100 days after exposure
- » Do not reintroduce Heparin as long as antibodies persist!

Anticoagulation

Coumadin (Warfarin)

- » Acts on extrinsic & common coagulation pathways
- » Monitor PT/INR
  - Normal PT = 11 - 13.5 sec
  - Normal INR = 0.8 - 1.1
- » Therapeutic goal INR 2 - 3
  - DVT Prophylaxis
  - PE Prophylaxis/treatment
  - Atrial fibrillation

- » Therapeutic goal INR 2.5 - 3.5
  - Mechanical prosthetic valves
- » To reverse warfarin:
  - Vitamin K (phytonadione) 2.5 - 5 mg PO
  - 1 - 2.5 mg IV SLOWLY over an hour
  - Will see INR drop within 8 - 12 hours

» **Serious or life threatening bleeding**

- Vitamin K 10 mg IV SLOWLY – never give IV push!
- Fresh Frozen Plasma (FFP)

- Prothrombin Complex Concentrate (PCC)
  ▷ K-Centra
  ▷ Often used with Vitamin K
- NovoSeven – recombinant factor seven

Heparin (unfractionated)

» **Acts on intrinsic & common coagulation pathways**

» **Monitor aPTT**

- Normal 25 – 38 seconds
- Can also monitor Factor Xa

» **For procedural sheath removal, can also monitor ACT**

- Therapeutic ACT 300 – 350 seconds
- Discontinue sheath when ACT < 150 seconds

» **Reversal: Protamine sulfate**

Protamine sulfate for anticoagulation reversal

» **Heparin reversal: 1 – 1.5 mg of Protamine per 100 units of Heparin**

- Do not exceed 50 mg Protamine IV

» **Dalteparin reversal: 1 mg of Protamine per 100 units of Dalteparin administered**

» **Enoxaparin reversal: 1 mg of Protamine per 1 mg of enoxaparin if enoxaparin given within 8 hours**

» **Adverse effects of Protamine:**

- Hypotension
- Nausea/vomiting
- Anaphylaxis
- Flushing
- May interact with NPH insulin, PCN or Cephalosporin antibiotics
- Anaphylaxis
  ▷ Fish allergies
  ▷ Protamine comes from salmon sperm

Low Molecular Weight Heparin vs. Unfractionated Heparin

Benefits of LMWH:

» Less incidence of HIT

» No need to monitor aPTT

» Longer half-life
  - 4 – 6 hours vs. 1 – 2 hours with UFH

» More predictable d/t bioavailability
  - 90% bioavailable vs. 30% with UFA

Direct Oral Anticoagulation (DOAC) – FYI only				
Drug:	**Works on:**	**Half-life:**	**FDA approval:**	**Reversal:**
Dabigatran (Pradaxa)	DTI, anti-factor IIa	12 – 17 hours	Non-Valvular afib, VTE Prophylaxis	Praxbind (idarucizumab)
Rivaroxaban (Xarelto)	Factor Xa inhibitor	7 – 11 hours	Non-Valvular afib, VTE prevention	Andexxa (Andexanet alfa)
Apixaban (Eliquis)	Factor Xa inhibitor	12 hours	Venous thromboembolic events	Andexxa (Andexanet alfa)
Edoxaban (Lixiana)	Factor Xa inhibitor	10 – 14 hours	VTE Prophylaxis after ortho surgery, stroke prevention	None available
Betrixaban (Bevyxxa)	Factor Xa inhibitor		VTE, DVT/PE (hospitalized patients)	None available

Neurology

Stroke

- » 5th leading cause of death in the US
- » Leading cause of disability
- » Hypertension is the biggest risk factor
  - Atrial fibrillation
  - Patent foramen ovale
- » Dysphagia is common & can lead to aspiration pneumonia

2 Types:

- » Ischemic
  - ~85% of all strokes
  - May present with transient ischemic attack (TIA)
  - TIA can be warning sign of stroke
  - Blood supply to brain tissue briefly halted
- » Hemorrhagic ~15%

AHA Stroke Guidelines

- » 1 hour goals:
  - Complete National Institute of Health Stroke Scale (NIHSS) Assessment
  - CT Scan without contrast
  - Glucose measurement
  - Treat with fibrinolytic therapy (if appropriate)
    ▷ Embolic only
  - Large vessel occlusions (LVO) benefit from thrombectomy

NIH Stroke Scale assesses:

- » LOC
- » Eye deviation (CN III, VI, VIII)
- » Visual field loss (hemianopia)
- » Facial palsy
- » Motor arms (drift)
- » Motor legs
- » Limb ataxia
- » Sensory

- » Language
- » Dysarthria
- » Extinction & inattention

- » Note: Higher score consistent with more severe stroke
  - Scores 0 - 42
  - Not a diagnostic tool

Diagnostics:

- » CT scan <u>without</u> contrast
  - R/O hemorrhage
  - Should be interpreted within 45 min
  - Might see hypodensity in ischemic area with ischemic stroke

- » CT perfusion or MRI perfusion
  - Measures infarct core or penumbra

Treatment: fibrinolytic therapy

Fibrinolytic considerations:

- » "Door to needle" time = 1 hour
- » Symptom onset window = extended 4.5 hour window, but shortened to 3 hours if:
  - Age > 80
  - Taking oral anticoagulation regardless of the INR
  - History of stroke & diabetes
  - Baseline NIHSS score > 25
- » Baseline labs/tests:
  - Glucose is the only requirement
  - CBC, coags, chemistry, troponin, 12 lead ECG are ideal

- » **Control BP prior to administration!!**
  - Goal SBP < 185, DBP < 110
- » rtPA (alteplase, activase)
  - Dosing: 0.9 mg/kg IV, max 90 mg
  - 10% of dose given over the 1st minute
  - The remaining infused over 1 hour
- » Tenectaplase (TNkase)
  - Dosing: 0.25 mg/kg (max 25 mg) bolus over 5 seconds
  - Increased affinity binding to fibrin
  - Less cerebral hemorrhage
  - Half-life ~ 20 min

Other medication tips:

- » If the patient received therapeutic doses of LMWH in the previous 24 hours, avoid rtPA
  - This does NOT include prophylactic doses!
- » Abciximab (Reopro) should NOT be administered concomitantly
- » Aspirin 325 mg should be given within 24 - 48 hours of stroke onset
- » Do not provide other anticoagulation therapy within 24 hours of rtPA
- » Begin statin therapy**
  - Restart statins if they were previously taking them

BP reduction strategies:

- » **Carefully** lower the BP
- » Avoid swings in BP!
- » BP goal:
  - ▷ < 185/110 before fibrinolytic is administered!
- » Which medications should be used?
  - ▷ Labetalol 10 – 20 mg IV over 1 – 2 min, repeat
  - ▷ Nicardipine 5 mg/hour IV, titrate up to 15 mg/hour max
  - ▷ Clevidipine 1 – 2 mg/hour, max 21 mg/hour
  - ▷ Hydralazine IV
  - ▷ Enalaprilat

Complications of rtPA include conversion to hemorrhage

- » **Conversion to ICH risk ~ 6%**
  - Some sources cite lower rates
- » **Symptoms:**
  - Deteriorating neuro exam
  - Headache
  - Nausea/vomiting
  - Acute hypertension

Other Patient Care Problems

» **Actions:**
- Prepare for STAT head CT scan
- Stat coags, fibrinogen, CBC

» **Prepare to transfuse if appropriate:**
- Platelets
- Cryoprecipitate
  ▷ Contains fibrinogen & clotting factors
- Tranexamic acid (TXA)
  ▷ Antifibrinolytic
- FFP
  ▷ Caution with the volume associated with administration!

Endovascular therapies for ischemic stroke:

» **Thrombectomy considered for large vessel occlusions (LVOs) within 24 hours of last known well**

» **Should receive rtPA regardless**

» **May be reasonable in patients with a contraindication to IV fibrinolysis**

» **Intra-arterial rtPA may also be considered**

Stroke care components:

» **Cardiac monitoring**
- Atrial fibrillation & cardiac arrhythmias
- TEE to assess for thrombus
  ▷ Left atrium & appendage often the culprit

» **Echocardigram**
- Assess for Atrial Septal Defect (ASD), Patent Foramen Ovale (PFO) or ventricular septal defect (VSD) as cause of stroke
- Bubble study

» **Restart anti-hypertensives after 24 hours**
- Should have specific BP target
- Higher target if no rtPA

» **Airway support**
- Ventilatory assistance if needed
- Apply O_2 if sats are < 94%
- Aspiration risk

» **Avoid fever!!! (temp > 37.5°C)**
- Antipyretic therapy
- Fever = ↑ morbidity & mortality

» **Treat hypovolemia**

» **Treat hypoglycemia (< 70 mg/dL)**
- Goal: normoglycemia
- BS 140 – 180
- Hyperglycemia is common as a neuroendocrine stress response
- Worse outcomes if hyper or hypoglycemic

- » **VTE prophylaxis**
  - Prophylactic anticoagulation &/or SCDs
  - Early mobilization
- » **NPO until swallow evaluation**
  - Nurse-driven swallow screen
  - If unable to take solids, consider placing a feeding tube
  - If > 2 weeks, consider PEG
- » **Avoid in-dwelling urinary catheters**
  - High risk of UTIs specifically in the neuro population

Nursing considerations for stroke care:

- » **Frequent neuro checks**
  - Monitor for signs of increased ICP
  - Placement of a Ventriculostomy drain if hydrocephalus develops
- » **Monitor for bleeding**
  - Conversion of embolic to hemorrhagic stroke
- » **Corticosteroids are not routinely recommended**
- » **Monitor for seizures**
  - Acute ischemic stroke is one of the highest causes of epilepsy in the elderly

Therapies to consider for stroke:

- » **Physical Therapy**
- » **Occupational Therapy**
- » **Speech**
- » **Long term placement if ongoing disability**
- » **Palliative Care if appropriate**
- » **Depression is common**

Carotid Stenosis

Clinical presentation:

- » TIAs, visual Δ's
- » Memory loss
- » Vertigo, syncope
- » Carotid bruit or thrill

Treatment:

- » Antiplatelet aggregation (ASA, Plavix)
- » BP control
  - Specific patient targets should be established
  - Do not want to lower too much
- » Carotid Endarterectomy
- » Carotid Stenting
- » Balloon angioplasty
  - Not done as much

Carotid Endarterectomy:

- » Post-op: Monitor for bleeding/hematoma
- » Close airway monitoring d/t location of incision
- » Regular neuro assessments post-op
- » Cranial nerve assessment:
  - VII: Smile
  - IX/X: Swallow, gag, speech
  - XI: Shrug shoulders
  - XII: Stick out tongue

Renal

Acute Kidney Injury (AKI)

- » Abrupt decline in glomerular filtration rate (GFR)
- » Results in retention of metabolic waste
  - Protein catabolism (azotemia)
- » Electrolyte & acid-base imbalance
- Retention of potassium, magnesium & phosphate
- Low calcium
- » Fluid overload
- » Acid/base imbalance
  - Metabolic acidosis

Causes of acute kidney injury:

- » Low perfusion, medications, parenchymal disease
- » Reversible if prompt treatment is received

Common laboratory evaluation in AKI:

- » Azotemia—elevated BUN
- » Elevated creatinine
  - Up to 12 hour lag time in elevation
    - ▷ Not an early indicator!
- » BUN/Creatinine ratio, normal ratio is 10:1 to 15:1
- » Glomerular Filtration Rate
  - Estimated by creatinine clearance
  - Normal is 80 – 120 ml/min
- » Urinalysis:
  - Casts - presence is a sign of tubular cell death
  - Electrolytes (specifically Na^+)
  - Albumin
  - Glucose
  - Protein

Prerenal AKI

- » Results from hypoperfusion
- » Kidney structure & function is preserved
- » Causes: Sepsis, heart failure, trauma, severe hypovolemia
- » BUN/Creatinine ratio > 20:1
  - BUN elevates, creatinine may start to elevate
- » Oliguria
- » Urine Na^+ < 20 mEq/L
  - Kidneys hold on to Na^+ & H_2O
- » Urine osmo & urine specific gravity ↑ due to concentration
- » HIGH RISK for progressing to ATN!

Treatment:

- » Treat cause, improve perfusion

Acute Tubular Necrosis (ATN)

- » May also be referred to "intrarenal" kidney injury
- » Injury occurs at the nephron; there is structural damage!
- » Causes: Hypotension, glomerulonephritis, diabetes, rhabdomyolysis, nephrotoxic medications, shock states
- » BUN > 25 mg/dL, creatinine > 1.2 mg/dL
- » BUN/Creatinine ratio 10:1
  - Both BUN & creatinine are elevated
- » Often requires renal replacement therapy (RRT)/dialysis

Treatment:

- » Depends on cause, assess if dialysis is indicated
- » Prevent & treat acidosis, electrolyte imbalance & uremia
- » Stop nephrotoxic medications
- » Ensure adequate cardiac output
- » Avoid NSAIDs!

Indications for Dialysis

Easy acronym to remember reasons:

- **A:** Acid/base imbalance
- **E:** Electrolyte imbalance (hyperkalemia, hypermagnesemia, hyperphosphatemia)
- **I:** Intoxications (ODs/toxins)
- **O:** Overload (fluid)
- **U:** Uremic symptoms

Laboratory findings in ATN in need of RRT:

- BUN > 35
- **Creatinine > 4 or, creatinine climbing ≥ 1 point/day**
- **Uncompensated metabolic acidosis**
- Anemia
- **Electrolyte imbalances**
  - Increased potassium (> 6.5), magnesium, phosphate
  - Decreased calcium, bicarbonate
  - Abnormal urine electrolytes

With all kidney injury, ensure patients:

1. Have adequate HYDRATION!
2. Have adequate PERFUSION!
3. Stop NEPHROTOXIC meds!

Uremic Syndrome Symptoms (when BUN is elevated)

» Neurologic: Lethargy, fatigue, seizures, coma

» Cardiovascular: ECG changes (d/t hyperkalemia), signs of fluid overload; tachycardia, S3 heart sound, hypo/hypertension

» Hematologic: Anemia

» Pulmonary: Crackles, pulmonary edema, SOB, effusions, pleuritis from uremia

» Gastrointestinal: Decreased appetite, nausea & vomiting, ascites & fluid overload

General Treatment Goals for AKI

» **Hemodynamic stability**

» **Improve renal perfusion**

» **Aggressive dialysis**

» **Correct chemistry abnormalities** (electrolytes, BUN, creatinine)

» **Monitor electrolyte imbalances**
- During & after dialysis

» **Adequate hydration**
- Careful use of diuretics
- Accurate, meticulous daily weights

» **Monitor drug levels for toxicity**

» **Monitor coags**

» **Alter medication schedules around dialysis if needed**

» **Modify medication dosing**—identify meds cleared through kidneys

» **Minimize exposure to nephrotoxic medications**

» **Prevent infection**

» **Maintain nutritional state**

Contrast induced nephropathy (CIN)

» **Highest risk patients:**
- Diabetics, HTN, heart failure
- Pre-existing renal insufficiency
- Dehydrated
- Concurrent use of nephrotoxic medications (i.e. NSAIDs, ACE Inhibitors)
- High volume of IV contrast
  ▷ 10% of all patients who receive contrast dye develop CIN—yikes!

» ***HYDRATION!!! is the key to prevention**
- A little rhyme to remember: The **solution** to **pollution** (contrast dye) is **dilution**!!!!
- Hydrate to protect the kidneys!!!

» **Sodium bicarbonate infusion— 1 hour before & 6 hours after exposure to contrast dye**
- Not much evidence to support this

» **N-Acetylcysteine (Mucomyst) for prevention (stinky!)**
- 600 mg PO day before & day of contrast exposure (total of 4 doses)
- Thought to prevent toxicity to renal tubules
- Not much evidence to support this

Dialysis

Hemodialysis

» **Intermittent**

» **Slow Low Efficiency Dialysis (SLED)**
- HD at lower flow rate; usually over 12 hours

» **Artificial kidney (hemofilter) with a synthetic membrane**

» **Dialysate is bicarbonate & sodium based with electrolytes**

» **Short term access**
- Double lumen catheter

» **Long term access**
- AV fistula

Hemodialysis Complications

- » Hypotension
- » Dysrhythmias
  - D/t electrolyte shifts
- » Angina
- » Fever from pyrogenic reaction
- » Coagulopathy, thrombocytopenia
- » Disequilibrium syndrome
  - Post-treatment cerebral edema
- » Air embolism (rare)

A quick acronym to remember medications removed by Dialysis:

- **B** - Barbiturates
- **L** - Lithium
- **I** - Isoniazid
- **S** - Salicylates
- **T** - Theophylline/Caffeine (both are methylxanthines)
- **M** - Methanol
- **E** - Ethylene glycol
- **D** - Depakote

Hold BP meds until after dialysis if appropriate!

Air Embolism

Venous signs:

- » Shortness of breath
- » Chest pain
- » Acute right heart failure
  - If obstructs blood flow from right heart to the lungs
- » Looks like a pulmonary embolism!

Treatment:

- » Lay on left side, trendelenburg position
- » Oxygenate with 100% O_2
  - Accelerates the removal of nitrogen in the air embolism
- » Hyperbaric oxygen therapy

Arterial signs:

- » Change in LOC (looks like a stroke!)
- » Decreased arterial flow & perfusion (looks like an occluded artery)
- » It only takes 2 ml of air to be fatal in an artery
  - Only 0.5 ml air to be fatal in a coronary artery

Treatment:

- » Oxygenate with 100% O_2

Continuous Renal Replacement Therapy (CRRT)

- » Slow continuous fluid removal
- » Used in patients who are hemodynamically unstable
- » Must have sufficient mean arterial pressure (MAP) or AV gradient to run CRRT
  - AV Gradient is calculated by using the MAP – CVP
  - \> 60 mm Hg is desired
- » If the AV gradient is too low, vasopressors may be needed to increase the blood pressure
- » Indications: fluid removal refractory to diuretics

Complications:

- » Hypotension
- » Bleeding (anticoagulation)
- » Hypothermia—can use a warmer
- » Filter/circuit clotting or clogging
- » Membrane rupture
  - Blood in effluent bag
  - Immediately stop treatment & disconnect!

CRRT modes

» Slow Continuous Ultrafiltration (SCUF)— removing excess fluid only

» Continuous venovenous hemofiltration (CVVH)
- With hemodialysis (CVVHD)
- With hemodiafiltration (CVVHDF)

Peritoneal Dialysis (PD)

» Primarily used for long term kidney failure, but can be used in emergencies

» Soft catheter inserted percutaneously into abdominal cavity

» Abdominal mesenteric capillary bed is utilized as the semi-permeable membrane

» Glucose-based dialysate is used
- 1.5%, 2.5%, 4.25% glucose solutions are often used
- 4.25% solution is going to pull more fluid off than 1.5%
- Higher glucose concentration = ↑ fluid removal via diffusion gradient

» Usually 2 liter exchanges done every 3 - 4 hours

» Advantages: patient can do at home, cost effective, no need for anticoagulation or vascular access

Complications of Peritoneal Dialysis (PD):

» Peritonitis
- Increased WBCs, temperature derangements

» Hyperglycemia

» Diaphragmatic pressure which can cause respiratory compromise

» Pleural effusions

» Visceral herniation or perforation

Contraindications to PD:

- Recent abdominal surgery
- Peritonitis
- Abdominal adhesions

Electrolyte Imbalances

Sodium

Functions:

- Regulates total body water
- Regulation of acid-base balance
- Transmission of nerve impulses
- Muscle contraction/cellular depolarization

Hypernatremia Na$^+$ > 145 mEq/L

Causes:

- Dehydration
- Hypertonic enteral feedings
- Excess administration of NaCl or NaHCO$_3$
- Burn injury

Symptoms:

- Thirst, tachycardia, hypotension, restless, irritable, lethargy, muscle weakness, flushed skin, oliguria (with dehydration)
- Increased serum osmolality
- Increased urine specific gravity due to concentrated urine in dehydration
  - Often > 1.025
- May also see increased hematocrit (hemo-concentrated)
- Decreased urine Na$^+$
  - May also see ↑ in absence of dehydration
- Chloride may be elevated as well
  - Often > 106 mEq/L

Treatment:

- Fluid hydration
- Free H$_2$O
- Diuretics (to remove sodium)—of appropriate for cause
  - Do **not** use if dehydrated

Hyponatremia—Na$^+$ < 130 mEq/L

Causes:

- Excess H$_2$O or Na$^+$ depletion
- Water retention
- Dehydration
- NG tube suction
- SIADH—dilutional hyponatremia
- Diarrhea
- Intestinal surgery
- DKA

Symptoms:

- Neuro changes, headache, confusion, coma, death
- Anxiety, weakness, abdominal cramping, seizures, hypotension, tachycardia, shock

Treatment:

Note: When treating hyponatremia, it's important to identify the patient's intravascular volume status:

1) Water retention/hypervolemia

- **Diuretics & sodium replacement may be administered**

2) Euvolemic

- **May only need to give sodium replacement**

3) Hypovolemia

- **May only need to give sodium replacement**

- » Slow Na⁺ correction!!!!
  - No more than 8 – 12 mEq/day
- » Na⁺ Phosphate 1 – 2 mmol/hour over 3 – 4 hours
- » Hypertonic saline
  - 2% or 3% infusion
- » Na⁺ tabs

Potassium

- » Normal K⁺ levels: 3.5 – 5.0 mEq/L
- » 98% intracellular, 2% in serum
- » Na⁺/K⁺ pump—maintains normal cell volume & electro-neutrality of the cell membrane

Functions of K⁺:

- » Transmission of nerve impulses
- » Intracellular osmolality
- » Enzymatic reactions
- » Acid-base balance
- » Myocardial, skeletal & smooth muscle contractility

Potassium Regulation

- » Kidneys—Primary excretory source
  - So efficient rarely have elevated states in normal renal function
  - In the presence of aldosterone, K⁺ is excreted by the renal tubules
- » Intestines—excrete K⁺

Hypokalemia: K⁺ < 3.5 mEq/L

Causes:

- » Increased loss
- » GI: Vomiting, NGT suctioning
  - Aggravated by metabolic alkalosis
- » Diarrhea, fistula, ileostomy
- » Excessive urinary loss
  - Hyperaldosterone states, thiazide diuretics, amphotericin, gentamycin, cisplatin

- » Inadequate intake
- » Anorexia, ETOH
- » Magnesium depletion
- » Insulin

Symptoms:

- » Clinical presentation—develop symptoms when K⁺ < 3.0 mEq/L
- » Cardiovascular irritability
  - Ventricular irritability (PVCs) K⁺ < 3.2
- » Ventricular fibrillation
- » Depressed ST segment
- » Development of u-wave

- » Prolonged QT interval
- » Potentates digoxin activity
- » Muscle cramping
- » **If the potassium is LOw, it causes Alka-LO-sis**
  - 0.1 unit ↑ in pH, causes ↓ K⁺ by 0.4 mEq/L

Treatment:

- » **Replace K⁺**
- » **Oral supplements or increased dietary intake when possible**

- » **IV - Standard dose 10 - 20 mEq over 1 - 2 hours**
  - Central line administration preferred
  - Dilute if giving through a peripheral IV

- » Eliminate or treat conditions that promote K⁺ shifts (i.e. alkalosis)

- » Ensure adequate renal function

Hyperkalemia - K^+ > 5.5 mEq

Causes:

- » Renal failure (~75% of all cases)
  - Inability of renal tubules to excrete K^+
- » Acidosis
- » Decreased cardiac output
- » Elderly taking K^+ sparing diuretics

- » Severe trauma & burns
- » Infection
- » Addison's disease
- » Increased consumption of table salt or antacids

Symptoms:

- » Nausea & vomiting
- » Diarrhea
- » Tingling skin

- » Numbness in hands & feet
- » Flaccid paralysis
- » Apathy, confusion

Cardiac symptoms:

- » Tall tented symmetrical T waves (K^+ > 6.5)
- » Widened QRS, prolonged PR, widened P wave (K^+ > 8.0)
- » Decreased automaticity (K^+ 10 - 11.0)
- » P waves disappear

- » QRS merges with the T wave to form sine wave
- » Asystole or ventricular fibrillation
- » Decreased strength of cardiac contraction

Treatment:

» **Emergency (move potassium):**

- Regular Insulin
  ▷ Dextrose if normal or low glucose to prevent hypoglycemia
- Nebulized albuterol
  ▷ Onset ~15 min., duration about 15 – 90 min.
- $NaHCO_3$—not as efficient as insulin
- Calcium chloride
  ▷ Cardiac protectant; no effect on K^+ levels

» **Remove potassium:**

- Dialysis
- Loop diuretics
- Sodium polystyrene sulfonate (Kayexalate)
  ▷ Dose 15 grams 1 - 4 doses/day
  ▷ 24 hours to correct
  ▷ Shouldn't be used for emergent treatment

Magnesium

» **Normal level 1.5 – 2.5 mEq/L**

Functions:

» **Neuromuscular transmission**

» **Cardiac contraction**

» **Activation of enzymes for cellular metabolism**

» **Active transport at the cellular level**

» **Transmission of hereditary info.**

Hypomagnesemia - Mg^{++} < 1.4 mEq/L

Causes:

- » **Increased excretion**
  - NG suctioning, diarrhea, fistulas
  - Diuretics: blocks Na$^+$ reabsorption
  - Osmotic diuresis
  - Antibiotics & anti-neoplastics
- » **Decreased intake**
- » **Chronic alcoholism**
- » **Malabsorption**
- » **Acute pancreatitis**

Symptoms:

- » **CV: Tachycardia, depressed ST segment**
- » **Torsades de Pointes! Caused by prolonged QT!**
  - Polymorphic ventricular tachycardia
- » **PACs & PVCs**
- » **Hypotension**
- » **Increased risk for digoxin toxicity**
- » **Coronary artery spasm**
- » **Neuromuscular**
  - Twitching, paresthesia, cramps, muscle tremors
  - + Chvostek & Trousseau's signs
    ▷ Twitching of face or hand
- » **CNS: mentation changes, seizures**
- » **Assess for hypokalemia**

Treatment:

- » **Assess renal function**
  - Reduce Mg^{++} replacement if renal dysfunction
- » **Increase Mg^{++} intake**
- » **Increased risk for digoxin toxicity**
- » **Dietary: diet or PO supplementation**
  - Add to IV or TPN

» MgSO$_4$ 1 - 2 grams IV over 60 minutes, <u>emergency</u> give over 1 - 2 minutes

- Give slowly if it's not an emergency
- Monitor BP & airway when administering magnesium!
- Can get hypotensive & flushed with Mg^{++}

» Monitor neurological status

» Monitor K$^+$ & Ca^{++}

» Follow serial magnesium levels

Hypermagnesemia - Mg^{++} > 2.5 mEq/L

Causes:

» Decreased excretion from renal failure is the most common

» Can also see in acidosis, DKA

Symptoms:

» 3 - 5 mEq/L Peripheral dilation, facial flushing, hypotension

» 4 - 7 mEq/L Drowsiness, lethargy

» When Mg^{++} is elevated, patients get the "Mag Drag"! (Lethargy, drowsy)

Treatment:

» Increase excretion of Mg^{++} by using fluids & diuretics

Hypocalcemia—Ca^{++} < 8.5

- » Follow ionized (active) Ca^{++}
- • Normal: 1.1 – 1.35 mmol/L

Causes:

- » Diarrhea
- » Diuretics
- » Malabsorption
- » Chronic renal failure

- » Alkalosis; Ca^{++} bound to albumin & is inactive
- » Phosphate & calcium have an inverse relationship to each other!
  - • ↑ PO_4 leads to ↓ Ca^{++}

Symptoms:

- » CV: Prolonged QTc, ↓ BP, ↓ CO, ventricular ectopy, ventricular fibrillation
- » Neuromuscular: Tingling, spasms, tetany, seizures
  - • Twitching, paresthesia, cramps, muscle tremors
  - • + Chvostek & Trousseau's signs

- » Respiratory: Bronchospasm; labored shallow breathing
- » Gastrointestinal: smooth muscle hyperactivity
- » Bleeding; Ca^{++} needed to clot
- » Safety: confusion & seizures
- » Muscle cramps can precede tetany

Treatment:

- » Administer calcium gluconate

Pulmonary

Arterial Blood Gases

Know the norms & review ABG interpretation for the CMC exam. I'm not going to do much in this book with ABGs.

Normal Blood Gas Values

pH:	7.35 - 7.45
PaO_2	80 - 100 on room air
$PaCO_2$	35 - 45
HCO_3	22 - 26
Base Deficit	-2 to +2
SaO_2	95 - 100%

If the pH is < 7.35 that leans toward acidosis, > 7.45 leans toward alkalosis

If the $PaCO_2$ is < 35 that leans toward alkalosis, > 45 leans toward acidosis

If the HCO_3 is < 22, that leans toward acidosis, > 26 leans toward alkalosis

Capnography—$PEtCO_2$

» Normal Capnography is 35 – 45 mm Hg

» Is a measure of ventilation, but also a reflection of perfusion & metabolism
- If cardiac output drops, capnography values will drop

» Continuous with waveform

» $PEtCO_2$ should be within 5 mm Hg of $PaCO_2$

» Is the gold standard method to verify endotracheal tube placement
- Lungs vs. gut...still need a chest x-ray to determine how high or low ET tube is

- » Standard of care for moderate to deep sedation
  - Hypoventilation = ↑ $EtCO_2$
  - Hyperventilation = ↓ $EtCO_2$
- » Used with PCA pumps to identify ineffective ventilation
- » Helpful to calculate deadspace & V/Q matching in certain conditions, like:
  - Pulmonary embolus
  - Pneumonia
  - Over-distention of alveoli from PEEP or tidal volume
  - Endotracheal tube in main stem bronchus
  - Asthma or COPD exacerbation
- » As a measure of perfusion, capnography is helpful with:
  - Resuscitation
    - CPR quality & ROSC
  - Low cardiac output states = low $PEtCO_2$
  - Correlation between $PEtCO_2$ & Cardiac Output
  - In cardiac arrest goal is > 10 mm Hg
- » Other uses:
  - Weaning the ventilator
  - Head injuries

Non-Invasive Positive Pressure Ventilation (NPPV)
CPAP/BiPAP

- » Continuous positive pressure
- » Stabilizes airways during exhalation
- » Improves ventilation (BiPap)
- » Keeps alveoli open
- » Used to treat:
  - COPD Exacerbation
  - CHF, pulmonary edema
  - Obstructive sleep apnea
  - Obesity hypoventilation syndrome
- » Monitor for facial skin breakdown

CPAP

» Simple mask & O_2

» Set at 5 – 10 cm H_2O

» Increases functional residual capacity
  • Volume in the lungs at end-exhalation

» Does not augment tidal volume

Bi-PAP

» Bi-level positive airway pressure

» CPAP that alternates between 2 pressure levels

» Higher mean airway pressures, more alveolar recruitment

» Provides larger tidal volumes

» Set IPAP & EPAP

» Typical starting point:
  • IPAP 10 cm H_2O, EPAP 5 cm H_2O
  • Inspiratory time 0.8 - 2 seconds

Acute Respiratory Distress Syndrome (ARDS)

» Inflammatory lung disease

» It is not a primary disease, but a result of:
  • Sepsis
  • Trauma
  • Multiple blood transfusions (TRALI, CRALI)
  • Pancreatitis
  • Cardiopulmonary bypass
  • Pulmonary contusion
  • Pneumonia/aspiration

What is happening in ARDS?

» INFLAMMATORY RESPONSE!

» Alveoli are infiltrated with leukocytes

» Widespread endothelial & alveolar damage
  • Leaky capillaries

» Lungs get stiff
  • Decreased compliance
  • Fibrin deposits in lungs

» Non-cardiogenic pulmonary edema

Signs:

- » Tachypnea
- » Progressive refractory hypoxemia
- » Worsening P/F ratio
  - $PaO_2 \div FiO_2$
  - Normal > 300
- » CXR—Bilateral pulmonary infiltrates
- » Usually require mechanical ventilation within 48 hours
- » Which therapies will improve the PaO_2?
  - Answer: PEEP & prone!

Diagnosis:

- » **Broncho-alveolar Lavage (BAL) or Bronchoscopy**
  - Sample examined for neutrophils & protein
  - Neutrophils: Up to 80% in ARDS
    - ▷ Normal: 5%
  - Higher protein level in aspirate, sign of inflammation
- » **Timing: within 1 week of a known clinical insult**
- » **Pulmonary infiltrates on CXR**
  - Bilateral opacities
- » **P/F ratio: < 300**

Berlin Criteria—2012

- » **P/F ratio:**
  - < 300—Mild ARDS
  - < 200—Moderate ARDS
  - < 100—Severe ARDS
- » **Predisposing conditions**
- » **Absence of left heart failure or left atrial hypertension**
  - Non-cardiogenic pulmonary edema
  - Mimics pneumonia & cardiogenic pulmonary edema

ARDS Treatment:

» **Rest the lungs**

» **Mechanical ventilation with "Lung Protective Ventilation" or "LPV"**

» **Low tidal volume**
- Start at 6 mL/kg PBW
- Lowest 4 mL/kg PBW

» **Larger tidal volumes over distend & rupture distal air space (volutrauma)**

» **Limit pressure related injury (barotrauma)**

» **Use predicted body weight when establishing tidal volume settings**

» **Use of PEEP**
- Think of PEEP as a stent to keep alveoli open

» **When increasing PEEP, monitor for signs of decreased cardiac output!!!**
- May see hypotension

» **Goal: End inspiratory plateau pressure < 30 cm H_2O**
- Inspiratory hold on the ventilator—measure pressure at that point
- If elevated, decrease the Vt

» **Allow permissive hypercapnia**

» **The goals aren't always to normalize the blood gas**
- Usually want pH > 7.2

Other therapies:

» **Conservative fluid management**
- Do NOT fluid overload patients!
- Diuretics
- Able to liberate the patient from the ventilator quicker!

» **Prone positioning**
- New evidence of benefit
- Must be done early, not rescue strategy
- Should remain prone > 16 hours per day

» **Inhaled pulmonary vasodilators**
- Epoprostenol (Flolan) or iNO (Nitric oxide)
- No evidence it improves outcomes
- Reduces pulmonary artery pressure
- Alleviates right heart strain

» **Optimize oxygen delivery**
- Cardiac output: Dobutamine
- PaO_2: PEEP
- Low hemoglobin: Only transfuse if necessary!

» **Neuromuscular blockade**
- For ventilator dyssynchrony

» **Extracorporeal Membrane Oxygenation (ECMO)**
- V – V ECMO
- Complete lung support

» **Steroids**
- No benefit from early steroids
- Some benefit days 7 – 14
- Methylprednisolone 2 – 3 mg/kg/day
- Inhibits fibrinolysis

Pulmonary Embolus

» **70% have a DVT**
- Usually from the deep venous system of the lower extremities

» **Alveoli are ventilated, but there is a lack of perfusion!**
- V/Q mismatch

» **Most emboli are multiple**

» **Lower lobes of lung are more commonly involved vs. upper lobes**

Risk factors:

» **Immobility*****

» **Surgery**

» **Trauma**

» **Clotting disorders**

» **Hemolytic anemia**

Signs:

- » Tachycardia
- » Tachypnea
- » Dyspnea
- » Chest pain
- » Crackles
- » Diaphoresis

- » Hemoptysis
- » Sudden right heart failure
- » Increased PA pressures
- » PEA Arrest
  - Dilated RV compresses LV

Diagnosis

- » Spiral (helical) CT scan—detector rotated around the patient; 2-D view
  - 30 seconds or less to perform scan
  - Hold breath at intervals during scan
  - Contrast infused to view pulmonary vasculature
  - 93% sensitivity / 97% specificity if clot is in one of the main arteries

Other diagnostics:

- » Pulmonary angiogram
  - Most accurate
  - Performed in < 20% of patients with PE because it takes too long
- » Ultrasound—DVT extremities
- » V/Q Scan—only diagnoses 25 – 30% of cases
  - Underlying lung disease—abnormal scan
- » Elevated Troponin = bad sign
- » 12 Lead ECG findings:
  - Not specific to PE
  - Right axis deviation
  - Transient right BBB
  - ST depression, T wave depression in $V_1 - V_4$
  - Tall peaked T waves in II, III, aVF
- » ABG—low PaO_2

Treatment:

If hemodynamically stable:

- » **Unfractionated Heparin (UFH)**
  - Weight-based dosing
  - Prevent progression
  - Bolus, then continuous infusion
  - Goal: aPTT 50 – 80 seconds
    - ▷ Some hospitals target 60 – 100 seconds

- » **Warfarin**
  - Used with UFH
  - Usually start on 1st day of Heparin therapy
  - Goal: INR 2 – 3, then d/c Heparin
  - Continue for 6 weeks

Can also use:

- » **Low Molecular Weight Heparin (LMWH)**
- » **Fondaparinux**

- » **Enoxaparin 1 mg/kg Q 12 hours**
  - Cleared by the kidneys (renal adjustment)
  - Simplified dosing
  - No need to monitor coags
  - Treat outpatient

- » **EKOS Catheter with rtPA**

If the patient has hemodynamic instability or cardiac arrest:

- » **Fibrinolytic therapy**
  - 12% chance of major hemorrhage
  - 1% ICH
  - Have to weigh benefit > risk

IVC Filters

Used for DVT if:

- » Contraindication to anticoagulation
- » Pulmonary embolus while on anticoagulation
- » Thrombus in right heart or free floating
- » No DVT, but ↑risk of hemorrhage

Pulmonary Arterial Hypertension (PAH)

- » High pressure in the pulmonary vasculature
  - Mean PAP ≥ 25 mmHg
- » Leads to right sided heart failure

Causes:

- » Idiopathic
- » Medications
- » Systemic hypertension
- » Obstructive sleep apnea (OSA)
- » Sclerotic diseases
- » Lung diseases

Common treatments for symptomatic PAH (oral):

- » Sildenafil (Viagra)
- » Bosentan (Tracleer)
- Both are pulmonary vasodilators

Rapid progression treatment:

- » Epoprostenol (Flolan) – Continuous IV (short half-life)
  - Always have an extra bag on standby
- » Treprostinil (Remodulin)
- » Goal with all meds is **pulmonary vasodilation**
- » Watch for hypotension

You Can Do It!

Quizzes with Answers & Rationale

Quiz 1 – Questions

1. The nurse is caring for a patient admitted with an inferior wall MI. On assessment, the patient has jugular venous distention with clear lung sounds. The vital signs are:

    HR 120

    BP 82/40 (54)

    RR 20

    SpO_2 95%

    The nurse anticipates which of the following orders?

    a. Isotonic fluid bolus

    b. Morphine sulfate IV push

    c. Lasix (furosemide) continuous infusion

    d. Metoprolol (Lopressor) 10 mg IV

2. The nurse preceptor is teaching a new nurse to perform transvenous pacemaker stimulation threshold testing at the beginning of the shift. Which statement would suggest to the nurse preceptor that additional education is needed?

    a. "Performing threshold testing at the beginning of the shift is an important safety measure."

    b. "It is important to explain to the patient and family why this needs to be performed and what they might experience."

    c. "The set point for the mA is the point at which capture resumes."

    d. "Before I start I need to ensure the patient is in a 100% paced rhythm."

3. The nurse is caring for a patient with ARDS who is intubated and mechanically ventilated. Patient data are as follows:

   HR 112

   BP 98/54 (68)

   SpO_2 86%

   CVP 4 mm Hg

   Cardiac Index 1.9 L/min/m²

   Ventilator settings:

   FiO_2 80%

   Ventilator set rate 22/minute

   Vt 6 mL/kg, volume mode

   PEEP +8

   The decision is made to increase the positive end expiratory pressure (PEEP) to + 12. What adverse effects in the patient hemodynamics should the nurse anticipate?

   a. Increase in the HR and decrease in the CVP

   b. Increase in the SpO_2 and increase in the BP

   c. Decrease in the HR and decrease in the CVP

   d. Decrease in the CVP and increase in the C.I.

4. A 56-year-old patient with a history of CAD (on aspirin & Plavix), Type II Diabetes & HTN arrives to the Emergency Department with a 3-day history of chest pain that is intermittent and worsens with activity. The 12 lead ECG reveals NSR with diffuse ST segment depression in 8 leads. The Troponin-I result is 5.5 mcg/L. The nurse anticipates the necessity of which intervention?

a. Cardiac catheterization

b. Chest CT Scan

c. Transesophageal Echo (TEE)

d. Chest x-ray

5. A patient with reduced EF (HFrEF) heart failure has a pulmonary artery catheter in place and is currently receiving Dobutamine (Dobutrex) at 7 mcg/kg/minute.

Current vital signs are:

HR 112

BP 98/62 (74)

RR 18

SpO_2 96%

C.O. 5.5 L/min

C.I. 2.9 L/min/m²

The nurse receives an order to decrease the Dobutamine (Dobutrex) infusion to 5 mcg/kg/min. How does the nurse know the dose change is tolerated by the patient?

a. A decrease in urine output

b. A decrease in the C.O.

c. An increase in heart rate

d. Urine output remains consistent

6. A patient is receiving a continuous heparin infusion for management of a NSTEMI. The patient notifies the nurse of sudden severe abdominal pain and the need to have a bowel movement. The nurse notes approximately 400 mls of frank-blood in the patient's stool. The heparin infusion is discontinued. The hematocrit level dropped from 38 to 26%. Which order should the nurse anticipate receiving next?

   a. Praxbind 2.5 grams IV

   b. Fresh frozen plasma (FFP) 2 units STAT

   c. Protamine sulfate 25 mg IV infusion

   d. Vitamin K (Phytonadione) 10 mg IV infusion

7. An ICU patient is being treated for unstable angina. The bedside monitor demonstrates new ST depression in lead II. A 12 lead ECG is obtained and is significant for ST segment elevation in V_1 - V_4 with reciprocal ST segment changes in II, III, & aVF. The nurse suspects:

   a. Anterior wall MI

   b. Posterior wall MI

   c. Lateral wall MI

   d. Inferior wall MI

8. A patient is admitted to the ICU with exacerbated systolic heart failure. The brain natriuretic peptide (BNP) level on admission is 1,593 pg/ml. The nurse understands which other laboratory value is necessary for interpretation of this result?

   a. Potassium

   b. Hematocrit

   c. Creatinine

   d. White Blood Cell (WBC)

9. When discussing risk factors for metabolic syndrome with a patient who is preparing for discharge, the nurse understands the patient's knowledge is correct when they describe which factors?

   a. Elevated blood pressure, increased waist circumference, elevated triglycerides

   b. Hyperglycemia, impaired renal function, elevated blood pressure

   c. Hyperglycemia, elevated total cholesterol, impaired renal function

   d. Hypokalemia, proteinuria, hyperglycemia

10. The nurse is preparing to administer TNKase (Tenecteplase) to a patient experiencing a ST elevation myocardial infarction (STEMI). Which order should the nurse question?

    a. Sequential compression devices to the bilateral lower extremities

    b. Insertion of an indwelling bladder catheter

    c. aPTT/INR/Fibrinogen every 6 hours

    d. Type & Screen (Crossmatch) for 2 units PRBCs

11. You admit a patient following coronary stent placement to the left circumflex artery. As the patient recovers, you notice the MAP has dropped from 68 mm Hg to 52 mm Hg with progressive variability in the systolic pressure tracing of the arterial line during inspiration & exhalation. The most likely explanation for this variability is:

    a. Suspected perforation in the left circumflex artery

    b. Post procedure pneumothorax

    c. A normal clinical finding following coronary stent placement

    d. Fluid overload

12. You observe that your patient with a transvenous pacemaker set to VVI is having pacer spikes within the QRS complex. The output is set at 5 mA and the sensitivity at 15 mV. Which of the following actions should you take first?

   a. Increase the sensitivity to 20 mV, making the pacemaker less sensitive

   b. Decrease the sensitivity to 8 mV, making the pacemaker more sensitive

   c. Decrease the output to 2 mA

   d. Increase the output to 10 mA

13. Your patient experienced a pulmonary embolism after a myocardial infarction. A heparin infusion was initiated. The morning CBC reveals a decrease in the platelet count by over 50% from her baseline count 4 days ago. What do expect as the next intervention?

   a. Repeat the CBC

   b. Transfuse platelets

   c. Stop the heparin infusion

   d. Send a HIT antibody test

14. You are caring for a patient with an IABP catheter in place on 1:1 ratio. You notice the urine output is dropping. A chest x-ray is obtained to confirm placement of the IABP catheter & tip. Correct positioning of the tip of the IABP lies at the:

   a. 1st to 2nd intercostal space

   b. 2nd to 3rd intercostal space

   c. 3rd to 4th intercostal space

   d. 4th to 5th intercostal space

15. Your patient admitted with chest pain is placed on the cardiac monitor. You notice the patient is in a heart block at a rate of 46 with a wide QRS complex. Some, but not all the atrial impulses are transmitted to the ventricles. There are frequent dropped ventricular complexes, but the PR interval is constant.

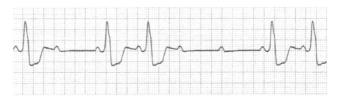

The type of block described is:

a. First Degree AV Block

b. Second Degree Type 1 AV Block

c. Second Degree Type 2 AV Block

d. Third Degree AV Block

16. Your patient is diagnosed with Wolf-Parkinson-White Syndrome (WPW). The two main clinical features of WPW include a shortened PR interval and a widened QRS complex with a delta wave. A delta wave is best described as:

a. A slurring in the upstroke of the QRS complex because of slow fiber to muscle fiber conduction

b. The point where the ST segment takes off from the QRS complex, which then becomes elevated due to early repolarization

c. A delay in conduction in the atrium, which manifests in the QRS complex due to the shortened PR interval

d. The point after the T wave when there is a small upward wave because of the delayed conduction in the ventricle

17. You are caring for a 72-year-old male diagnosed with an inferior wall MI. He has acute complaints of SOB and tachypnea. When auscultating heart sounds you discover a high pitched, holosystolic murmur radiating to the axilla, best heard at the apex. Which of the following complications do you suspect?

    a. Papillary muscle rupture

    b. Aortic Regurgitation

    c. Pericarditis

    d. Aortic Stenosis

18. A patient with a history of systolic heart failure is admitted with signs of shock. A pulmonary artery catheter is placed to evaluate cardiac function and intra-cardiac filling pressures. Hemodynamic findings are as follows:

    HR 100 bpm

    BP 110/80 (90)

    SpO_2 97%

    C.O. 3.2 L/min

    C.I. 1.8 L/min/m²

    RAP 16 mm Hg

    PA 46/24 mm Hg

    PAOP 20 mm Hg

    SvO_2 40%

    SVR 1886 dynes/sec/cm^{-5}

Based on this hemodynamic profile, a Dobutamine infusion was initiated. Which of the following medications should be used in addition to Dobutamine to manage this patient?

a. Nitroglycerin & Dopamine infusions

b. Milrinone & Norepinephrine infusions

c. Sodium Nitroprusside (Nipride) infusion & furosemide (Lasix) IVP

d. Furosemide (Lasix) IVP & Dopamine infusion

19. A patient with severe systolic dysfunction is being discharged from the hospital after re-admission for volume overload. Spironolactone was started prior to hospital discharge. Which of the following best describes the action of this medication as it relates to the treatment of heart failure with systolic dysfunction?

a. Slows conduction through the AV node decreasing myocardial oxygen demand

b. Vasodilates smooth muscle decreasing the work load on the heart

c. Slows development of hypertrophy and fibrosis of the myocardium

d. Improves LV function by aiding in the retention of serum potassium

20. You are caring for a patient with infective endocarditis of the aortic valve. Blood cultures are positive for *S. Aureus*. Which of the following choices would achieve the best possible patient outcome?

a. A full course of antibiotics prior to cardiac surgery

b. IV antibiotics and immediate surgical debridement

c. Immediate trans-catheter aortic valve replacement

d. Antibiotics until blood cultures are negative, then proceed with surgery

Quiz 1 - Answers

1. A. Isotonic fluid bolus. Patients experiencing an inferior wall MI often become preload dependent. The stunned right ventricle can cause a significant decrease in ventricular output from the RV, thereby decreasing forward flow to the left side of the heart. Maintaining preload and contractility of the right ventricle is important.

Isotonic fluids will increase preload and promote forward flow of blood from the right to left side of the heart. If the patient remains unstable, a Dobutamine infusion may be considered. Lasix, beta-blockers & morphine all reduce preload by either decreasing volume, decreasing contractility, or vasodilating and should be avoided.

2. C. "The set point for the mA is the point at which capture resumes." The set point for the mA after threshold testing needs to be 2 - 3 times the mA when capture is restored. This is done to provide a safety margin. For example, if capture is regained at 2 mA, the set point mA for safety is at least 4 mA - 6 mA.

3. A. Increase in the HR and decrease in the CVP. As the PEEP is increased, the pressure in the thoracic cavity increases. In turn, venous return to the right atrium can decrease resulting in decreased cardiac output. A decrease in HR would not be anticipated with an increase in PEEP. While an increase in SpO_2 is expected with an increase in PEEP, a decrease in venous return with a decrease in BP would be anticipated with this ventilator change. Not every patient is going to experience these hemodynamic changes, but you should be prepared to intervene if needed. If the BP drops with PEEP changes, simply decrease the PEEP to the level prior to the increase & reassess the BP.

4. A. Cardiac catheterization. Cardiac catheterization is appropriate as the patient is high risk with a history of CAD on dual anti-platelet therapy, presenting with a NSTEMI and elevated cardiac biomarkers. Visualization of the coronary arteries is the anticipated investigative assessment.

5. D. Urine output remains consistent. Dobutamine is a strong, positive inotropic agent. With a decrease in the dosage, a decrease in C.O./C.I. and urine output is possible and may occur. A significant drop in urine output may require an increase in the Dobutamine infusion dose. The patient's response to weaning Dobutamine should be closely monitored for signs of decreased perfusion.

6. C. Protamine sulfate 25 mg IV infusion. Protamine sulfate is the reversal agent for acute heparin overdoses. Protamine sulfate is dosed 0.5 mg – 1.5 mg/100 units depending on the time from heparin administration. The maximum dose of Protamine sulfate is 50 mg. Higher doses of Protamine can create a paradoxical effect and cause bleeding.

Administer IV slowly over 10 minutes. Overdosing or rapid administration of Protamine sulfate can cause hypotension, cardiovascular collapse (related to hypotension), non-cardiogenic pulmonary edema, pulmonary vasoconstriction and pulmonary hypertension. For hypersensitivity reactions (coughing, wheezing, hives, & edema), IM-epinephrine should be readily available.

Protamine sulfate should be avoided in patients with fish allergies as it is derived from salmon sperm (not sure who figured that one out!). Also, it may interact with penicillin or Cephalosporins.

7. A. Anterior wall MI. ST elevation in precordial leads with reciprocal changes in the inferior leads is significant for an anterior wall MI. Further risk for septal or lateral wall damage is a concern. Assessment for development of systolic murmurs, signs and symptoms of heart failure, shock, and changes in the ECG rhythm including heart blocks is important. The patient should be loaded with aspirin and emergently taken to the Cardiac Catheterization Lab.

8. C. Creatinine. The BNP peptide is cleared through the kidneys, therefore a creatinine value is contributory for guiding interpretation with an elevated BNP. This value can be interpreted as mild-moderate heart failure. A BNP level < 100 pg/ml is interpreted as normal; heart failure or overstretching of the ventricle is not present. BNP > 100 pg/ml is interpreted as heart failure with overstretch of the ventricles. Clinical judgement is always necessary for interpretation.

9. A. Elevated blood pressure, increased waist circumference, elevated triglycerides. Insulin resistance, increased waist circumference, elevated triglycerides and HTN are significant components of metabolic syndrome. These criteria are known as "The Deadly Quartet". Renal function, hypokalemia & proteinuria are not identified risk factors for metabolic syndrome.

10. B. Insertion of an indwelling bladder catheter. Venous and arterial punctures and placement of invasive devices should be avoided for 24 hours after administration of a fibrinolytic. Oscillometric BP cuffs should be used with extreme caution due to the high exertional pressure. There is risk of bleeding because of the constant and frequent high-pressure compression cycling.

SCDs exert very little pressure on the extremities. The nurse should expect to monitor labs. A Type & Screen is expected in the event transfusions are required.

11. A. Suspected perforation in the left circumflex artery. Stent edge dissections are rare; only 6.6% per lesion. A perforated coronary artery following (PCI) is rare, but can lead to pericardial tamponade if not treated immediately. Following percutaneous coronary intervention (PCI), if patients are going to develop bleeding & cardiac tamponade from dissection, 50% will develop it within 10 - 20 minutes of stent deployment. Over 33% of patients with a dissection will develop tamponade 1 - 2 hours following PCI.

A sign of pericardial tamponade is Pulsus paradoxus. Normally during inspiration, the systolic blood pressure varies < 10 mm Hg, and is typically not detectable by palpation of the peripheral pulse. A decrease in systolic blood pressure > 10 mm Hg with inspiration is known as Pulsus paradoxus. Pericardial tamponade should be suspected and immediately evaluated in this scenario.

12. B. Decrease the sensitivity to 8 mV, making the pacemaker more sensitive. A pacing stimulus delivered during ventricular repolarization can be dangerous and lead to life threatening ventricular arrhythmias if it was delivered during the relative refractory period. A pacer spike within the QRS is indicative the pacer is not sensing or "seeing" ventricular activity and inhibiting the pacer to deliver a pacing stimulus. Therefore, it is not sensitive enough to identify the patient's intrinsic rhythm. The sensitivity value/setting (mV) needs to be evaluated and decreased.

13. C. Stop the heparin infusion. Discontinuation of the heparin infusion is the most appropriate initial intervention. Heparin Induced Thrombocytopenia (HIT) can cause life threatening thrombosis and bleeding. Results from antibody/assay testing can take several days to result. Since continued anticoagulation is required, a Direct Thrombin Inhibitor like Argatroban or Bivalirudin should be used.

14. B. 2nd to 3rd intercostal space. Low urine output may be an indication of malposition of the IABP catheter due to occlusion of the renal arteries. To maintain optimal blood flow to subclavian artery and renal arteries, the tip must lie between the 2nd to 3rd intercostal spaces. The balloon catheter should be distal to the left subclavian artery and superior to the renal arteries.

15. C. Second Degree Type 2 AV block. In a 2nd Degree Type 2 AV Block, the PR interval is constant, except when the electrical signal does reach the ventricles causing depolarization.

In a 2nd Degree Type 1 AV Block (Wenckebach) there is progressive lengthening in conduction through the AV node (varying PR interval) and intermittent conduction does not make it through to the ventricles.

In Third Degree AV Block, impulses are not reaching the ventricles to stimulate depolarization. Second degree heart block type 2 and complete heart block often require emergent pacing.

16. A. A slurring in the upstroke of the QRS complex because of slow fiber to muscle fiber conduction. In WPW, the QRS complex is widened because of premature ventricular action (vs. delayed in a bundle branch block). Most of the ventricular myocardium is activated through the normal pathway. However, there is a small area that is depolarized early and gives the QRS complex a slurred initial upstroke called a delta wave.

17. A. Papillary muscle rupture. Mitral regurgitation or papillary muscle rupture would be identified by hearing a high pitched holosystolic murmur, radiating to the axilla and best heard at the apex. Papillary rupture can occur acutely in the setting of a myocardial infarction. Patients with inferior/posterior MIs are at increased risk.

18. C. Sodium Nitroprusside (Nipride) infusion & furosemide (Lasix). The hemodynamic profile is consistent with cardiogenic shock. This is likely due to volume overload as evidenced by an elevated RAP & PAOP. The patient is in a low cardiac output state with increased afterload.

When the kidneys are poorly perfused, there is an increase in angiotensin II, which acts as a potent arterial vasoconstrictor resulting in an elevated SVR. This hastens blood flow from a failing left ventricle. Initiation of an arterial vasodilator will lower the SVR, and improve forward blood flow from the left ventricle. It will also augment diuresis by improving blood flow to the kidneys.

Nitroglycerin would be a less favorable choice given that it is a strong venous vasodilator and less of an arterial vasodilator. Dobutamine & Milrinone may also be considered if the C.O. remains low following diuresis & afterload reduction.

19. C. Slows development of hypertrophy and fibrosis of the myocardium. Spironolactone and Eplerenone are mineralocorticoid receptor antagonists (MRA) that have demonstrated a significant reduction in mortality when combined with other standard heart failure medications. Side effects include hyperkalemia and gynecomastia (less with Eplerenone).

Aldosterone is produced within a diseased heart, and has been shown to cause fibrosis and arrhythmias. Spironolactone blocks the effects of aldosterone on the heart by binding to the mineralocorticoid receptors on the heart. Potassium levels should be closely monitored, especially if Spironolactone is combined with an ACE Inhibitor or ARB.

20. B. IV antibiotics and surgical debridement. The AHA/ACC guidelines were updated in 2017 with no changes to the management of IE (infective endocarditis). There is a IIb recommendation for early surgical debridement and replacement of the valve without completing a full course of antibiotics when the suspected organism is *S. Aureus* and it is on the left side of the heart (aortic or mitral valve).

In general, high dose IV antibiotics are initiated to optimize the diffusion of antibiotics into the vegetations. Depending on the cause and bacteria, antibiotics are used for a 2 – 6 week course.

Right sided IE is less common and is often due to IV drug abuse. Left sided IE is more common and can be caused by IV drug injections and nosocomial in patients with prosthetic valves.

Quiz 2 - Questions

1. The nurse is reviewing the CVP tracing of a patient with severe tricuspid regurgitation. Which finding in the CVP tracing would be expected?

    a. Peaked c waves

    b. Enlarged v waves

    c. Flattened a waves

    d. Absent v waves

2. A patient returns from the Cardiac Catheterization Lab after dual chamber pacemaker placement. The settings on the pacemaker indicate the ventricles are paced, sensing occurs in the atria and ventricles, and atrial sensing triggers ventricular pacing while ventricular sensing inhibits ventricular pacing. The nurse documents this pacing mode as:

    a. DDD

    b. VDD

    c. DDI

    d. DVI

3. The nurse is admitting a patient with a history of heart failure being treated for septic shock. The patient is intubated and a pulmonary artery catheter is placed.

    Patient data:

    HR 125

    BP 82/40 (54)

    T 35.5° C

    SpO_2 90%

CVP 4 mm Hg
C.O. 2.9 L/min
C.I. 1.7 L/min/m²
SvO_2 40%

pH 7.16
$PaCO_2$ 38
PaO_2 80
HCO_3 18
Lactate 11 mmol/L

The primary goal of initial treatment includes:

a. Lowering the heart rate to < 80 bpm
b. Raising the CVP to 14 mm Hg
c. Improving oxygen delivery to tissues
d. Correcting acid/base imbalance with a sodium bicarbonate infusion

4. A patient is admitted with chest pain and shortness of breath. The patient describes severe 8/10 chest pressure. The 12 lead ECG shows ST depression in the anterior and inferior leads. The Troponin-I is 3.5 mcg/L. Which order does the nurse anticipate prioritizing?

a. Aspirin 325 mg chewable STAT
b. Metoprolol (Lopressor) 12.5 mg oral
c. Amlodipine 5 mg PO
d. Morphine 2 mg IV push

5. A patient is admitted for presumed septic shock from bacterial endocarditis. The patient presents with an alteration in mental status, cool extremities and jugular venous distension. The patient is started on a continuous infusion of Norepinephrine and Dobutamine (Dobutrex). The patient is also started on high dose IV antibiotics and the Cardiac Surgery team is consulted.

   Patient vital signs are as follows:

   HR 98

   BP 74/36 (49)

   RR 20

   SpO$_2$ 92%

   The nurse understands treatment is effective based on which assessment parameters?

   a. Improved capillary refill time & increased urine output
   b. Increased oxygen saturation & decreased HR
   c. Increased SBP & no change in urine output
   d. Decreased MAP & increased urine output

6. A patient admitted to the ICU after an antero-septal wall MI has developed acute dyspnea, crackles on auscultation, S3 heart sound and a new, loud holosystolic murmur. The nurse suspects:

   a. Tricuspid regurgitation
   b. Mitral regurgitation
   c. Papillary muscle rupture
   d. Ventricular septal rupture

7. A patient admitted with a hypertensive emergency has been on Nitroprusside (Nipride) for 48 hours. The current infusion dose is 3.5 mcg/kg/hour to be titrated to maintain the SBP < 165 mm Hg. The patient is alert and oriented, following commands. Current vital signs are as follows:

> HR 115
>
> BP 182/94 (123)
>
> RR 20
>
> SpO_2 95% on room air
>
> Which order should the nurse anticipate?

   a. Stop Nitroprusside (Nipride) & transition to Nicardipine (Cardene) at 5 mg/hour

   b. Continue Nitroprusside (Nipride) & administer Metoprolol (Lopressor) 5 mg IV push

   c. Send a Methemoglobin level STAT

   d. Continue Nitroprusside (Nipride) & increase the dose

8. A patient admitted to the ICU for cardiogenic shock has been on bedrest for six days. The nurse notes a sudden decrease in oxygen saturations. The FiO_2 is increased without a noted increase in oxygen saturation. The patient is extremely anxious and is coughing up blood-tinged secretions through the endotracheal tube (ETT).

> A chest x-ray is performed and is negative. An arterial blood gas (ABG) is then obtained.

   HR 130

   BP 124/60 (81)

   RR 32

   T 36.8° C

   SpO_2 86%

   $PEtCO_2$ 23 mm Hg

ABG results:

pH 7.28

$PaCO_2$ 60

PaO_2 50

HCO_3 24

Ventilator settings:

FiO_2 85%

Rate 20

Vt 450

PEEP +12

Which of the following conditions should be suspected?

    a. Pulmonary hypertension

    b. Pneumothorax

    c. Pulmonary embolism

    d. Cardiac tamponade

9. A patient arrives to the Emergency Department with severe 8/10 chest pain. A 12 lead ECG demonstrates ST elevation in the anterior and lateral leads. During cardiac catheterization the coronary arteries appeared open, but there was significant ballooning of the left ventricle. The patient was prepared for a Transesophageal ECHO (TEE). Which condition does the nurse suspect?

    a. Ventricular hypertrophy

    b. Pericarditis

    c. Pulmonary embolism

    d. Takotsubo Cardiomyopathy

10. A patient with a history of intravenous substance abuse is admitted for treatment of infective endocarditis (IE). They have developed a new systolic murmur, S3 ventricular gallop, dyspnea, and crackles in the bilateral lung bases.

> Vital signs:
>
> T 39.0° C
>
> BP 152/90 (111)
>
> HR 110
>
> RR 32
>
> SpO_2 92%
>
> The nurse should anticipate:

a. Intravenous furosemide (Lasix) and 25% albumin

b. Furosemide (Lasix) and intravenous morphine sulfate

c. Intravenous Nitroglycerin and furosemide (Lasix)

d. Beta blockers and a heparin infusion

11. In which of the following leads would you expect to see changes resulting from left circumflex coronary artery plaque rupture causing a STEMI with posterior wall involvement?

a. ST elevation in V1, V2, V3, V4, V5, and V6

b. ST depression in V1, V2, and V3

c. Unable to evaluate with an ECG

d. ST depression in lead III and aVF

12. A 28-year-old patient with history of anxiety, depression and ETOH abuse is admitted for a heroin overdose. She is now extubated, restless and agitated, complaining of pain and nausea. Her BP and HR are elevated. Which of the following medications would prompt a baseline 12 Lead ECG prior to administration?

    a. Clonidine

    b. Ativan

    c. Haldol

    d. Oxycodone

13. You are caring for a patient who experienced a cardiac arrest with a hypoxic-ischemic brain injury. The patient is placed on a ventilator liberation protocol. He is currently on pressure support at 3 cm H_2O, PEEP +5, FiO_2 30% with tidal volumes ranging from 120 ml to 500 ml & respiratory rates of 30 – 35 bpm. The SpO_2 is > 96%. The ventilator is occasionally alarming for low minute ventilation. You call the Respiratory Therapist and should suggest which of the following?

    a. Extubate the patient

    b. Increase the pressure support setting to 10 cm H_2O

    c. Assess the endotracheal tube for a cuff leak

    d. Increase the PEEP level setting

14. Your patient has a Pulmonary Artery Catheter in place and is having frequent runs of V-Tach. You notice that the PA waveform shows the following tracing:

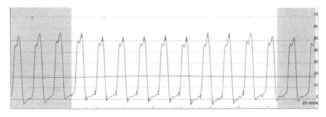

Your immediate action is to:

a. Reposition the patent to their left side

b. Ensure there is a blood return and re-zero the PA line

c. Ensure balloon is deflated and advance the catheter to the pulmonary artery

d. Ensure the balloon is deflated and pull back the catheter to the right atrium

15. A 56-year-old patient experienced a ventricular fibrillation cardiac arrest. In the middle of the second round of CPR the PEtCO$_2$ suddenly goes from 20 to 45 mm Hg. What is the next action to take?

a. Administer Epinephrine 1 mg IV

b. Increase the assisted ventilation rate to 20 breaths/min

c. Continue CPR until the next pulse check, the patient likely has ROSC

d. Assess for equal bilateral breath sounds

16. A 75-year-old female is admitted with exacerbated heart failure. She appears disengaged and confused. You suspect she may be developing delirium. When talking with her family about her delirium, the most appropriate statement is:

a. "At her age, we expect delirium to occur while she is in the hospital. Once her heart failure is treated, it will go away."

b. "Her heart failure is causing her to be confused. We can give her a medication to treat the delirium."

c. "Delirium can occur in situations like this. We will treat her heart failure and try to promote normal activities as much as possible."

d. "She is older and at higher risk to be confused in the hospital. I'm sure it will resolve when she goes home."

17. An 80-year-old female with systolic heart failure (HFrEF) is admitted with shortness of breath. Four months ago, her ejection fraction was measured at 34%. Your assessment of her notes shortness of breath, inability to lie flat, or speak in complete sentences. She is 20 pounds above her baseline weight and has significant peripheral edema. Her other complaints include lack of appetite, nausea, tense feeling in her abdomen and fatigue.

A central line was placed in the ED prior to being transferred to your unit. She was given 40 mg of Lasix IV 3 hours prior and has diuresed 200 mL. Her creatinine was noted to be 2.2 mg/dl and BNP was 3500 pg/mL.

> Vital signs:
>
> HR 110 bpm in Sinus Tachycardia
>
> BP 100/50 (66)
>
> RR 30
>
> O_2 saturations of 92% on 5 liters nasal cannula
>
> What should be anticipated in her plan of care?

    a. Continue monitoring, her creatinine is too high to give any more Lasix at this time

    b. Give a dose of Lasix at 40 mg PO because that is what she takes at home

    c. Start a Dopamine infusion, titrate to keep MAP > 65 mm Hg

    d. Assess a $ScvO_2$ & administer Lasix 80 mg IV

18. A 68-year-old female experienced a ventricular fibrillation cardiac arrest. Upon successful resuscitation, the patient is transported to the Emergency Department. Patient history is significant for coronary artery disease, dyslipidemia, and hypertension. The initial 12 Lead ECG is shown below:

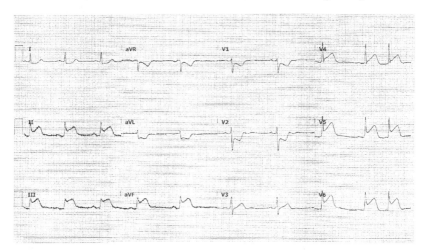

Which wall of the heart is likely experiencing an active myocardial infarction?

a. Anteroseptal

b. Anteroseptal & Lateral

c. Inferior & Lateral

d. Inferoposterior & Lateral

19. Which of the following patients is at highest risk of developing Contrast Induced Nephropathy?

a. 56 year old male with GFR of 60 mL/min and serum creatinine of 1.3

b. 70 year old diabetic female with GFR of 35 mL/min and serum creatinine of 1.2

c. 70 year old diabetic male who received 75 mL of contrast 5 days ago

d. 80 year old female with a GFR of 60 mL/min and serum creatinine of 2.0

20. You are caring for a patient who was admitted with an inferior wall myocardial infarction. Which of the following is a potentially fatal complication of an inferior wall MI?

   a. Ventricular septal rupture

   b. Papillary muscle rupture

   c. Hemopericardium

   d. Mitral valve prolapse

Quiz 2 – Answers

1. B. Enlarged v waves. Tricuspid regurgitation occurs when blood leaks backward into the right atrium with contraction of the right ventricle. It is often related to pulmonary HTN & other conditions causing high pressure on the right side of the heart. The enlarged v wave (also known as "canon waves") on the CVP tracing is seen because of increased volume and pressure on the right side of the heart and regurgitant blood flow into the right atrium.

2. B. VDD. When reading the letters of pacemaker modes, it is necessary to know the code. The first letter describes the chamber that is paced (A= atrium, V= ventricle, D= dual). The second letter describes the chamber where intrinsic activity is sensed (A= atrium, V= ventricle, D= dual), and the third letter describes the pacemaker's response to sensing (I= inhibit, T= trigger, D= dual). A pacemaker in VDD mode senses the atria and ventricles, but paces only the ventricles. It can both inhibit and trigger impulses based on the sensing.

3. C. Improving oxygen delivery to tissues. Oxygen delivery and perfusion are compromised as indicated by a low cardiac index and significantly low SvO_2. Fluids, vasopressors and positive inotropic support (i.e. Dobutamine) may be included in the initial medical management to improve oxygen delivery and tissue perfusion.

4. A. Aspirin 325 mg chewable STAT. Aspirin administration is a priority for anyone with UA/ NSTEMI & STEMI. Aspirin inhibits platelet activation and aggregation through the irreversible inhibition of cyclooxygenase (COX) and prevents the synthesis of prostaglandins. Aspirin is indicated for its mechanism of action in an NSTEMI. Nitrates & morphine will also be a consideration for comfort and pain relief. Oxygen should only be administered if the O_2 sats are < 94%.

5. A. Improved capillary refill time & increased urine output. This patient is presenting with a hypodynamic shock appearance. Assessing the signs of improved tissue perfusion as well as improved mental status, urine output & adequate BP is essential. Septic shock has both hyperdynamic and hypodynamic presentations.

Hyperdynamic septic shock (the "warm" stage) is characterized by high cardiac output, hypotension, low systemic vascular resistance (SVR) due to vasodilation & decreased SvO_2. These all may be reflective of inadequate resuscitation or severe vasodilation.

Hypodynamic septic shock (the "cold" stage) also presents with hypotension, metabolic acidosis and an increased SVR. The SvO_2 is often elevated because capillary micro emboli prevent oxygen delivery to the tissues, resulting in decreased oxygen extraction. The SvO_2 will be high as oxygen cannot get extracted to the tissues. Mortality in the hypodynamic state is extremely high.

6. D. Ventricular septal rupture. Rupture of the ventricular septum presents emergently as fluid overload with hypoperfusion. If a pulmonary artery catheter is in place, an increased C.O., increased SvO_2, and large v waves in the CVP waveform may be visible. This is related to the blood shunting from the left ventricle to the right ventricle. However, in reality, the cardiac output isn't actually elevated, it is very low. A pulmonary artery catheter may falsely interpret a high cardiac output because the C.O. sensor is located in the right ventricle. It will read an erroneously high C.O. because of the left to right shunting. The SvO_2 is truly elevated, because oxygenated blood is shunting from the left to the right.

Papillary muscle rupture is mostly seen in inferior wall myocardial infarctions. Valvular regurgitation may be present for a number of different reasons.

7. A. Stop Nitroprusside (Nipride) & transition to Nicardipine (Cardene) at 5 mg/hour. With increasing doses of Nipride and decreasing effectiveness, tachyphylaxis is possible and it will be important to switch medications. Most common adverse effects include direct vasodilation resulting in hypotension and dysrhythmias.

Higher doses put a patient at risk for toxicity. Signs include tinnitus, altered mental status, nausea, & abdominal pain. Cyanide toxicity can occur, but is rare. It can result in coma, metabolic acidosis or respiratory arrest. Methemoglobinemia is also rare, but can occur.

Toxicity is usually related to prolonged administration or occurs in patients with renal or hepatic failure.

Nicardipine is safest as a calcium channel blocker that is selective to vascular smooth muscle. Administration of IV push Metoprolol will not likely impact or minimize the dose and possible side effects.

8. C. Pulmonary embolism. For an intubated patient, refractory hypoxemia is significant diagnostic criteria for pulmonary embolism (PE). Other possible PE clinical presentation symptoms include: anxiety, hemoptysis, crackles, chest pain, increased PA pressures and in extreme cases PEA/cardiac arrest.

Comparison between $PEtCO_2$ and $PaCO_2$ can be useful in the diagnosis of pulmonary embolism. The combination of low CO_2 transport and poorly perfused lungs that are ventilated (dead space), leads to a decrease in expired CO_2 and an increasing difference between arterial and alveolar CO_2. This creates ventilation/perfusion (V/Q) mismatch. The arterial CO_2 levels will rise, while exhaled CO_2 drops.

9. D. Takotsubo Cardiomyopathy. Referred to as "broken heart syndrome" or "stress induced cardiomyopathy", Takotsubo is believed to be caused by a surge in stress hormones (catecholamine). Takotsubo is reversible and almost exclusively affects women greater than 55 years old. On echocardiogram, a ballooning left ventricle is often visible and can sometimes resemble an hourglass shape.

10. C. Intravenous nitroglycerin and furosemide (Lasix). The most common complication of infective endocarditis (IE) is heart failure as a result of valvular insufficiency. Medical management prioritizes diuresis and afterload reduction for heart failure development and pulmonary edema.

While morphine provides afterload reduction, a more appropriate medication for the development of acute mitral regurgitation is Nitroglycerin. It can be used in conjunction with diuresis and ACE inhibitors.

11. B. ST depression in V1, V2, and V3. An occlusion of the left circumflex artery (LCx) can affect the posterior wall of the heart. Therefore, ST depressions in V1 through V3 are reciprocal changes, and to accurately evaluate a posterior infarct you would need to obtain a posterior ECG. These ECG changes may also be seen with a lesion in the RCA. If a patient has left dominant coronary circulation (10% of the population) then the inferior wall is supplied via the LCx and PDA. In these patients, an occlusion of the LCx would also result in inferior ECG changes (leads II, III & aVF).

12. C. Haldol. A patient with history of Heroin use is at risk for a prolonged QT interval. Haldol can also prolong the QT interval. A baseline 12 Lead ECG with a calculated corrected QT interval should be assessed prior to administering Haldol.

This patient may be experiencing withdrawal symptoms. Clonidine can be used to depress sympathetic tone & response. A benzodiazepine may be used to help with anxiety and restlessness. Oxycodone, while not first line treatment for opioid withdrawal, will help with symptoms this patient is experiencing. None of these medications prompt the need for a baseline 12 Lead ECG.

13. B. Increase the pressure support setting to 10 cm H_2O. A pressure support setting of 3 cm H_2O is minimal to assist the patient in overcoming the resistance of the endotracheal tube & possible airway swelling while spontaneously breathing. Increasing the pressure support will provide additional assistance to alleviate respiratory workload, hopefully leading to decreased respiratory rate and increased tidal volumes. If this does not work, the patient may need to be placed back onto controlled mechanical ventilation.

14. D. Ensure the balloon is deflated and pull back the catheter to the right atrium. The PA tracing waveform indicates the catheter tip is located in the right ventricle. If the patient is experiencing ventricular ectopy, this could progress to a life-threatening emergency. After ensuring the balloon is deflated, the catheter must be withdrawn within the sterile sleeve until a right atrial tracing is visible.

15. C. Continue CPR until the next pulse check, the patient likely has ROSC. While the $PEtCO_2$ has dramatically improved during CPR, it is still essential to continue chest compressions for the full cycle. A rapid rise in the $PEtCO_2$ is likely a sign of return of spontaneous circulation (ROSC).

16. C. "Delirium can occur in situations like this. We will treat her heart failure and try to promote normal activities as much possible." Delirium puts patients at higher risk for increased hospital length of stay and mortality. Treating the underlying cause of delirium is key to prevention & progression. Providing normalcy such as night/day routine, sleep hygiene, ensuring she has glasses & hearing aids, engagement in activities & exercise are just a few things that will improve symptoms of delirium.

17. D. Assess a $ScvO_2$ & administer Lasix 80 mg IV. This patient has exacerbated heart failure. She has over distension of the ventricle and managing her worsening heart failure symptoms are priority. A low $ScvO_2$, less than 70%, demonstrates hypo-perfusion in the setting of excess fluid.

Lasix is a loop diuretic and should be doubled when its effects are minimal. In an exacerbated patient, Lasix should be administered IV. The $ScvO_2$ should improve with Lasix administration. If she continues to have signs of heart failure, a positive inotrope like Dobutamine or Milrinone may be considered.

18. **D. Inferoposterior & Lateral.** Leads II, III, and aVF view the inferior wall of the left ventricle. Leads V_5 and V_6 view at the low lateral wall of the left ventricle. In all of the aforementioned leads, there is the pattern of ST segment elevation indicative of myocardial injury. In the presence of Inferior MI, ST segment depression in leads V_1 and V_2 with tall R-waves may indicate acute posterior wall MI as well. The ST depression in leads V_1 and V_2 represents a reciprocal change. If leads were placed directly below the left scapula (giving a direct view of the posterior wall), they likely would reveal ST elevation.

19. **B. 70 year old diabetic female with GFR of 35 mL/min and serum creatinine of 1.2.** Patients identified as highest risk for CIN (contrast induced nephropathy) are those with a GFR < 45 mL/min and the presence of proteinuria, diabetes, dehydration or other comorbid conditions. For patients with a GFR < 30 mL/min, it is recommended to administer pre-and post-treatment intravenous fluids. Hydration is the key to prevention of CIN!

Administration of acetylcysteine (oral or IV) is no longer recommended. In a recent publication there was no benefit to using sodium bicarbonate and acetylcysteine for prophylaxis or treatment.

20. **B. Papillary muscle rupture.** Papillary muscle rupture is most common with an inferior wall MI due to the posterior papillary muscle's single blood supply of the posterior descending artery (PDA). The size of the myocardial infarct does not correlate to the incidence of papillary muscle rupture post infarction. When the papillary muscle ruptures, acute mitral regurgitation can lead to cardiogenic shock, pulmonary edema and death.

Quiz 3 – Questions

1. A patient with an anterior wall MI experiences a sudden rhythm change. The patient is lethargic & diaphoretic. A weak, thready pulse is palpable. The ventricular rate is noted to be 30 beats per minute, BP 68/46. P waves are present, but are not associated with the QRS complexes. The priority in treating this patient includes:

    a. Send serum Troponin and CK-MB

    b. Obtain a 12 Lead ECG

    c. Prepare Epinephrine for administration

    d. Emergent transcutaneous pacing

2. A patient is admitted to the ICU with an implanted dual chamber pacemaker and assessment of pacemaker function is prioritized. The presence of a P wave after every atrial pacing spike as well as the presence of a QRS complex after every ventricular pacing spike is verified to assess capture. The nurse utilizes which method to determine the AV delay?

    a. Assessing for intrinsic ventricular activity

    b. Measuring the interval between atrial pacing spikes in sequentially paced beats

    c. Measuring the interval from the atrial to ventricular spike in AV sequentially paced beats

    d. The presence of a P wave followed by a QRS complex

3. The nurse is called to the bedside of a 40-year-old patient with sharp 8/10 chest pain that came on suddenly while they were sleeping. As the nurse prepares to obtain a 12 lead ECG and draw a serum Troponin-I, the patient states the chest pain is subsiding. Prinzmetal's angina is suspected in this patient. Which of the following is the highest priority?

a. Obtain a chest x-ray

b. Obtain a 12 Lead ECG and repeat with recurrent chest pain

c. Administer Metoprolol (Lopressor)

d. Administer 325 mg Aspirin

4. A patient presents to the Emergency Department with blurred vision, severe headache and significant confusion.

Vital signs:

HR 102

BP 230/132 (165)

RR 24

T 37.2° C

The nurse anticipates which of the following orders?

a. Sublingual Nitroglycerin 2 tabs now

b. Nitroglycerin 20 mcg/min continuous infusion

c. Nicardipine 5 mg/hour continuous infusion

d. Labetalol 10 mg IV push every 5 minutes x 2

5. The nurse is caring for a patient admitted with right-sided heart failure and fluid overload. The monitor alarms and a rapid, regular rhythm is noted.

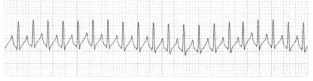

The patient is alert, sitting in bed and denies chest pain.

Vital signs are as follows:

HR 180 & regular

BP 108/62 (77)

RR 18

SpO$_2$ 96%

What is the appropriate first action to take?

a. Administer 500 mL lactated ringer's bolus

b. Apply defibrillation pads & charge the defibrillator to 200 joules

c. Have the patient cough & bear down

d. Administer Adenosine (Adenocard) 6 mg rapid IV push

6. The nurse is caring for a patient who is 3 days post myocardial infarction. Patient vital signs are as follows:

HR 90

BP 120/54 (76)

RR 28

SpO$_2$ 98% on 2 L NC

T 38.4° C

The patient describes slight mid-sternal chest pain. A 12 lead ECG shows slight ST elevation in leads II, aVR, and V$_2$ - V$_6$. On assessment, a pericardial friction rub is auscultated and the patient describes pain that worsens with coughing and position changes. The nurse should anticipate which of the following orders?

a. Aspirin 325 mg STAT chewed

b. Heparin continuous infusion

c. Chest CT scan STAT

d. Ibuprofen 800 mg PO

7. In addition to aspirin and a P2Y$_{12}$ inhibitor, which of the following medications should be anticipated to be initiated in your patient who is hemodynamically stable, but experienced an acute anterior/septal wall MI with mild left ventricular failure and stent placement to the LAD?

   a. ARB, calcium channel blocker & high dose statin
   b. Calcium channel blocker, beta blocker & aldosterone antagonist
   c. High dose statin, beta blocker & ACE inhibitor
   d. Beta blocker, ARB & aldosterone antagonist

8. A patient with an IABP placed 1 week ago has developed a petechial rash in the bilateral lower extremities. The patient has been receiving a Heparin infusion for a diagnosed deep vein thrombosis (DVT). A complete blood count (CBC) is sent. Current results are as follows:

   WBC 12.5
   Hgb 7.5 g/dl
   HCT 22%
   Platelet count 57,000 per microliter

   Which medication order should the nurse anticipate?

   a. Bivalirudin (Angiomax)
   b. Alteplase (Activase)
   c. Warfarin (Coumadin)
   d. Enoxaparin (Lovenox)

9. A patient is admitted with presumed Cardiomyopathy to the ICU. A pulmonary artery catheter is in place. The nurse assesses crackles in bilateral bases, tachypnea, audible S3 and a wet, non-productive cough. From this description, which of the following hemodynamic parameters would be expected?

a. CVP 14 mm Hg, C.I. 1.6 L/min/m^2, PA 46/24 mm Hg, PAOP 20 mm Hg

b. CVP 16 mm Hg, C.I. 2.6 L/min/m^2, PA 40/22 mm Hg, PAOP 8 mm Hg

c. CVP 2 mm Hg, C.I. 2.0 L/min/m^2, PA 20/8 mm Hg, PAOP 6 mm Hg

d. CVP 10 mm Hg, C.I. 3.5 L/min/m^2, PA 22/12 mm Hg, PAOP 12 mm Hg

10. The nurse is caring for a patient admitted with septic shock who has a history of systolic heart failure. A pulmonary artery catheter is placed to determine cardiac function & fluid responsiveness related to hemodynamic instability.

Vital signs:

HR 130

BP 88/40 (56)

SpO$_2$ 95% on 4 L NC

CVP 2 mm Hg

C.I. 4.5 L/min

SVR 386 dynes/sec/cm^{-5}

ScvO$_2$ 48%

The nurse should anticipate which of the following orders?

a. Intravenous crystalloid and Norepinephrine infusion

b. Intravenous crystalloid and Dopamine infusion

c. 100% FiO$_2$ and metoprolol (Lopressor) IV push

d. Dobutamine infusion and 2 units PRBC transfusion

11. A 70-year-old patient who is who had an ablation is being recovered in the post procedure observation area. He calls out and says, "Something isn't right, I can't breathe." He is diaphoretic with pale and clammy skin. His pulse rate is 118 in a sinus tachycardia rhythm. The BP is 74/68 (70). Considering the patient's complaint and physiologic data, which of the following conditions do you suspect following his ablation?

    a. Pulmonary embolism

    b. Pneumonia

    c. Pericardial tamponade

    d. ST Elevation Myocardial Infarction

12. You admit a 60-year-old female with a history of systolic heart failure. An Echocardiogram was performed revealing an EF 32%. Which of the following medications would you expect to be a part of the initial treatment?

    a. Metoprolol 25 mg BID

    b. Amlodipine 5 mg daily

    c. Captopril 6.25 mg TID

    d. Digoxin 0.125 mg daily

13. A 31-year-old female with a history of heart failure is being treated for metastatic cervical cancer. She has a serum calcium level of 16 mg/dL. You expect which of the following symptoms?

    a. Hypertension, muscle spasms, confusion

    b. Hypotension, muscle weakness, renal insufficiency

    c. Hypertension, bradycardia, nausea and vomiting

    d. Hypotension, tachycardia, nausea and vomiting

14. The best statement to describe how Amiodarone works as an antiarrhythmic is as follows:

    a. It blocks potassium channels and slows outward movement of potassium during phase 3 of action potential (rapid repolarization)

    b. It stabilizes the cell membrane by binding to sodium channels, depressing phase 0 of action potential (beginning of cell stimulation)

    c. It blocks calcium channels throughout action potential, completely shortening it

    d. It blocks the beta receptor sites causing a depression of phase 4 of action potential (cell rest)

15. Which of the following hemodynamic scenarios indicate the need for a Dobutamine infusion & diuretics?

    a. C.I. 1.7, CVP 2, PAOP 6, SVR 1950

    b. C.I. 2.2, CVP 6, PAOP 8, SVR 700

    c. C.I. 2.6, CVP 8, PAOP 10, SVR 1500

    d. C.I. 1.8, CVP 12, PAOP 16, SVR 1800

16. Which of the following medications is contraindicated after a myocardial infarction?

    a. Aspirin

    b. Metoprolol

    c. Multivitamin

    d. Ibuprofen

17. A 73-year-old male presents to the hospital with a complaint of chest pain and shortness of breath. The Troponin-I level is elevated. The 12 lead ECG shows the following:

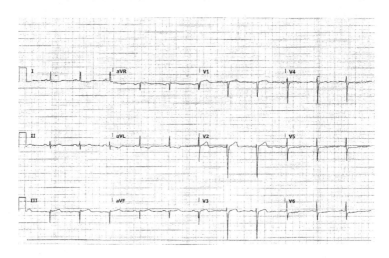

Based on the 12 Lead ECG results, which wall of the heart has infarcted and experienced damage?

a. Anterior

b. Anteroseptal

c. Inferior

d. Lateral

18. A patient with systolic heart failure is readmitted with shortness of breath & malaise.

Labs:

BNP 1,035 pg/mL

Ferritin 50 ng/mL

Sodium 132 mEq/L

Based on the lab values, which of the following do you anticipate the provider to order?

a. Lasix for diuresis
   b. Iron replacement therapy
   c. Cardiac Rehabilitation
   d. Increase beta blocker dose

19. In review of left and right ventricular pressure waveforms for a patent diagnosed with constrictive pericarditis, you would expect which of the following?
   a. Discordance of the LV and RV systolic pressures with respiration
   b. Concordance of the LV and RV systolic pressures with respiration
   c. Equalization of LV and RV systolic pressures
   d. Presence of the dip and plateau sign or "square root sign"

20. Amiodarone is a common antiarrhythmic used to treat atrial fibrillation. Which side effect associated with long-term use would prompt immediate discontinuation of the drug?
   a. Nausea & vomiting
   b. Cornea micro deposits
   c. Hypothyroidism
   d. Pulmonary fibrosis

Quiz 3 – Answers

1. D. Emergent transcutaneous pacing. The rhythm change is complete heart block and the priority is to restore cardiac output. The patient is severely symptomatic with bradycardia & hypotension. Complete heart block is significant because of the loss of conduction of atrial impulses to ventricles. Contraction of the atria and ventricles is dissociated. This dissociation leads to a loss of atrial kick, loss of atrial filling, and the slow ventricular rate decreases cardiac output significantly. Transcutaneous pacing is short-term intervention to restore cardiac output and increase the ventricular output. A transvenous or permanent pacemaker would need to be placed for more stable or long-term treatment.

2. C. Measuring the interval from the atrial to ventricular spike in AV sequentially paced beats. The AV delay is the setting that mimics the PR interval. It is the amount of time between sensed or paced atrial events and ventricular pacing output (the time period between the atrial and ventricular paced beats). Assessing for intrinsic activity will assess sensitivity. Measuring the interval between atrial spikes will determine the minimum pacing rate. A P wave followed by a QRS complex indicates a normal electrical cardiac cycle.

3. B. Obtain a 12 Lead ECG and repeat with recurrent chest pain. Variant (Prinzmetal's) angina occurs at rest. It is treated with Nitroglycerin and calcium channel blockers. Obtaining a 12 Lead ECG with and without chest pain is important to assess for ST segment changes associated with possible coronary artery vasospasm. ECG changes visible in Prinzmetal's angina include transient ST segment elevation with attacks of chest pain.

4. C. Nicardipine 5 mg/hour continuous infusion. This patient is presenting with a hypertensive emergency and signs of hypertensive encephalopathy. Clinical signs include blurred vision, headache, and confusion.

Calcium channel blockers are the preferred medication in a hypertensive emergency. Nicardipine is selective for vascular smooth muscle and is a direct arterial vasodilator. The goal is to reduce the MAP no more than 25% in the first 8 hours.

Sublingual medication is inappropriate treatment for HTN emergency, but may be considered in hypertensive urgency. Nitroprusside can be considered, but has significant toxicity effects and risks.

5. C. Have the patient cough & bear down. As the patient is not acutely unstable it is important to begin with Valsalva interventions of coughing and bearing down to stimulate the vagus nerve (parasympathetic stimulation). If the rhythm does not slow, adenosine can be administered starting with 6 mg and repeated doses of 12 mg.

Defibrillation would not be indicated, as it is used for pulseless rhythms. If the patient becomes unstable, synchronized cardioversion may be performed. Fluids should be given cautiously as the patient may not tolerate it due to the tachycardia and go into heart failure.

6. D. Ibuprofen 800 mg PO. The patient has developed acute pericarditis. Fever & non-specific ST segment changes may be noted, as well as a pericardial friction rub. Patients often report worsening pain with position changes and with coughing. There may be relief with sitting up & leaning forward. First line treatment includes NSAIDs to minimize inflammation and the inflammatory response. Antibiotics would be appropriate if the pericarditis was bacterial in origin and antivirals are appropriate if viral. Neither aspirin nor heparin is indicated for pericarditis.

7. C. High dose statin, beta blocker & ACE inhibitor. Beta blockers are a highly prioritized medication after a myocardial infarction. They have numerous short and long term benefits. Those include arrhythmia protection, decreasing contractility and automaticity as well as slowing myocardial remodeling longer term. In addition, beta blockers decrease the workload of the heart. Statins also have numerous benefits that include a decreased recurrence of MI & stroke as well as lowering lipids and providing anti-inflammatory benefits. ACE inhibitors are prioritized in any patient with a reduced EF of less than or equal to 40%. In addition, an aldosterone antagonist like spironolactone or eplerenone will likely be added to the regimen.

8. A. Bivalirudin (Angiomax). Bivalirudin is a Direct Thrombin Inhibitor and is an alternative for anticoagulation for patients with HIT. Heparin induced thrombocytopenia is an immune mediated adverse drug reaction caused by antibodies that develop after exposure to heparin. Platelets become activated placing patients at risk for the development of thrombosis.

9. A. CVP 14 mm Hg, C.I. 1.6 L/min/m^2, PA 46/24 mm Hg, PAOP 20 mm Hg. The clinical presentation matches left-sided heart failure. The expected hemodynamics would be decreased cardiac output with elevated CVP, pulmonary artery and pulmonary artery occlusive pressures. In addition, the systemic vascular resistance (SVR) will be elevated.

10. A. Intravenous crystalloid and Norepinephrine infusion. The patient data highlights hypovolemia and inadequate tissue perfusion with a ScvO$_2$ of 48% as a measure of oxygen extraction. The hyperdynamic state requires fluid and vasopressor administration to improve tissue perfusion. The low SVR demonstrates vasodilation expected in the warm or "hyperdynamic" stages of sepsis.

11. C. Pericardial tamponade. This patient is exhibiting signs of shock related to acute cardiac tamponade. Pericardial tamponade is a potential risk after an ablation due to myocardial perforation. Signs of pericardial tamponade include: tachycardia as a compensatory mechanism for low cardiac output, Pulsus paradoxus and narrow pulse pressure. Pulse pressure = SBP minus DBP. Normal pulse pressure is 40 mm Hg (120 – 80). This patient's pulse pressure is 6 mm Hg, which is considered "narrow" and consistent with pericardial tamponade.

It is essential to notify the provider emergently and prepare for urgent treatment to reduce the pericardial pressure. A chest x-ray, Transthoracic Echo (TTE) and pericardiocentesis should be anticipated.

12. B. Captopril 6.25 mg TID. Heart failure with reduced ejection fraction is known as HFrEF or Systolic Heart Failure. The initial line of treatment includes aggressive diuresis with loop diuretics and initiation of ACE inhibitors. ACE Inhibitors provide more rapid hemodynamic benefit and will not exacerbate HF in the short run.

The rapid improvement in hemodynamics that can occur with ACE Inhibitors may facilitate the subsequent initiation of beta blockers, which may transiently impair hemodynamics and symptoms. The patient likely will be discharged on an ACE-Inhibitor or ARB, beta blocker and an aldosterone antagonist like spironolactone.

13. B. Hypotension, muscle weakness, renal insufficiency. The normal serum concentration of calcium is 8.5 - 10.2 mg/dL. Patients with severe hypercalcemia (> 14 mg/dL) can exhibit symptoms including muscles weakness, dehydration, anorexia, nausea and vomiting and changes in sensorium, bradycardia, hypertension, shortened QT interval.

14. A. It blocks potassium channels and slows outward movement of potassium during phase 3 of action potential (rapid repolarization). Amiodarone is a Class 3 Antiarrhythmic which blocks potassium channels and slows outward movement of potassium during phase 3 of action potential prolonging it.

15. D. C.I. 1.8, CVP 12, PAOP 16, SVR 1800. Dobutamine is a positive inotrope and is utilized to augment cardiac output. An added benefit of Dobutamine is vasodilation. This often leads to a reduction in afterload or systemic vascular resistance (SVR) & will decrease the workload of the left ventricle. It should be used cautiously in patients that are not adequately volume resuscitated as this can cause arrhythmias. Given the high CVP & PAOP, hypovolemia is unlikely the case in this scenario. If Dobutamine is administered to a patient that is hypovolemic, it can cause hypotension.

16. D. Ibuprofen. Nonsteroidal anti-inflammatory medications (NSAIDS) are contraindicated and should be discontinued immediately. NSAIDs (except for aspirin), should not be administered during hospitalization for STEMI because of the increased risk of mortality, re-infarction, hypertension, heart failure and myocardial rupture associated with their use.

17. C. Inferior. The pathologic Q-waves Leads III and aVF demonstrate an infarct pattern in the inferior wall of the left ventricle. The positive Troponin-I level in the absence of ST-segment elevation is indicative of NSTE-ACS.

18. B. Iron replacement therapy. In 2017 the AHA/ACC/HFSA published a focused update to the heart failure guidelines. In this update, they focused on treatment of anemia, and specifically iron deficiency anemia. For patients who meet the following profile (Ferritin < 100 ng/ml, or 100 - 300 ng/ml and have a transferrin saturation < 20%), there is a IIb recommendation to treat with intravenous iron replacement therapy. Positive outcomes reported include an increase in exercise capacity, quality of life, BNP and left ventricular ejection fraction. It is not recommended to treat with erythropoietin stimulating agents (level of evidence III).

19. A. Discordance of the LV and RV systolic pressures with respiration. In patients with constrictive pericarditis, the amount of the blood within the heart is fixed due a stiff pericardium. The noncompliant pericardium does not allow the heart to relax completely, thus causing diastolic pressures to increase. Changes in intrathoracic pressures associated with respiration also create pressure differences. Normally with inspiration the right ventricular volume increases and left ventricular volume decreases. In the setting of a noncompliant pericardium, ventricular interdependence is observed. During inspiration RV systolic pressure decreases while LV systolic pressure increases; a classic finding of constrictive heart disease.

20. D. Pulmonary fibrosis. Pulmonary fibrosis is one of the most serious side effects of Amiodarone use. This may result in an abnormal chest x-ray and pulmonary function tests. Amiodarone should be discontinued and the patient treated with steroids.

Hypothyroidism is easily managed with levothyroxine and not cause for discontinuation. Cornea micro deposits are not associated with impairment of visual acuity with Amiodarone use.

Quiz 4 – Questions

1. A patient with a temporary transvenous pacemaker is set in VVI mode. The nurse observes the presence of pacer spikes immediately after an intrinsic ventricular contraction. Which action by the nurse is appropriate?

    a. Decrease the sensitivity (mV) value

    b. Increase the mA

    c. Increase the sensitivity (mV) value

    d. Perform a threshold test

2. A 58-year-old with an anterior wall MI is being treated with an Intra-aortic balloon pump (IABP). On initial assessment, the nurse is reviewing the augmentation waveforms. To ensure proper timing, the nurse verifies:

    a. Balloon inflation should occur prior to the dicrotic notch

    b. Timing of deflation should be done to avoid the lowest pressure possible

    c. An elevated systolic pressure following balloon deflation

    d. Balloon inflation occurs at the dicrotic notch and deflation at end diastole

3. A patient arrives to the Emergency Department with severe chest pressure. A 12 lead ECG reveals ST segment depression in the inferior and anterior leads. What additional data confirms the diagnosis of NSTEMI?

    a. Troponin-I of 1.5 mcg/L

    b. CK 55 u/L

    c. ST depression in aVR

    d. Relief of chest pain with administration of NSAIDs

4. The nurse is preparing a patient for discharge with a new diagnosis of hypertension. Which of the following patient statements signals to the nurse that additional education is required?

    a. "Losing weight will be the biggest contributor to reducing my blood pressure."
    b. "I will join a walking group with the parks department."
    c. "As long as I am exercising, having a few drinks every day is ok."
    d. "I will start reading the nutrition labels and tracking my sodium intake."

5. The Rapid Response Team is called to the CT scanner for a patient who suddenly became unresponsive. On arrival, chest compressions are in progress because a pulse was not palpable. What is the highest priority & intervention to provide to a pulseless patient?

    a. Provide assisted ventilations
    b. Apply defibrillation pads and turn on the defibrillator
    c. Verify the absence of a pulse without CPR
    d. Administer 1 mg Epinephrine IV push

6. A patient arrives to the Emergency Department complaining of light-headedness, nausea, and back pain. Vital signs on arrival:

    HR 50
    BP 82/50 (61)
    RR 18
    T 36.4° C

    The 12 lead ECG shows ST segment elevation in II, III & aVF with reciprocal lead changes in I & aVL. The nurse suspects:

a. Posterior wall MI

b. Anterior wall MI

c. Inferior wall MI

d. Septal wall MI

7. A patient with Cardiomyopathy has been on bedrest with limited activity tolerance for three days. The patient notifies the nurse of pain and decreased sensation in their right leg. The nurse anticipates which of the following orders?

   a. D-Dimer & fibrinogen levels

   b. Complete blood count (CBC)

   c. Chest x-ray

   d. Doppler ultrasound

8. The nurse is caring for a patient receiving a continuous heparin infusion after diagnosis of pulmonary embolism (PE). The nurse assesses a petechial rash across the chest and bilateral flanks. What is the appropriate priority by the nurse?

   a. Send a complete blood count (CBC)

   b. Perform a guaiac stool test

   c. Send coagulation studies

   d. Send STAT liver function tests

9. The nurse has completed wedging a pulmonary artery catheter and blood is visible in the syringe of the balloon port. After notifying the provider, what urgent action should the nurse anticipate?

a. Discontinuation of the pulmonary artery catheter

b. STAT chest x-ray

c. Advancement of the catheter

d. Echocardiogram

10. A patient with a pulmonary artery catheter is repositioned to their left side. The nurse observes a change in the PA waveform. The PA pressure values have changed from 38/18 to a mean value of 35 mm Hg. The waveform has changed and the dicrotic notch is no longer visible. After repositioning the patient to their back, the waveform has not changed. What is the priority of the nurse?

   a. Inflate the balloon and advance the catheter until a wedge waveform is observed

   b. Order a STAT Chest x-ray and basic metabolic panel

   c. Ensure the balloon is deflated and pull back until a PA waveform is observed

   d. Flush the catheter and zero and level the transducer

11. An 88-year-old female admitted to your unit with syncope. She is placed on the monitor and her cardiac rhythm initially reveals Second Degree Heart Block Type 2 (Mobitz II). She puts her call light on and states that she is not feeling well. You assess her cardiac rhythm and realize she is now in Complete Heart Block. Her heart rate is 34 bpm and blood pressure is 78/46 (56) and she is getting confused. What is your initial priority?

   a. Prepare to give atropine 1 mg IVP

   b. Initiate fluids wide open

   c. Prepare to transcutaneous pace

   d. Administer Epinephrine 1 mg IVP

12. You admit a patient on an ACE Inhibitor with a potassium level of 6.2 mEq/L. In addition to the ACE Inhibitor, which of the following medications could be contributing to the hyperkalemia?

   a. Sildenafil

   b. Spironolactone

   c. Amlodipine

   d. Theophylline

13. A 70-year-old patient s/p fall with multiple rib fractures and a pulmonary contusion is ventilated on Assist Control mode, Rate 16, FiO_2 70%, PEEP + 10. Her tidal volumes are ranging from 350 - 500 mls with a RR of 28 - 32. She is having frequent desaturation events.

   ABG results:

   pH 7.31

   $PaCO_2$ 54

   PaO_2 60

   HCO_3 24

   The patient is experiencing which of the following?

   a. Metabolic acidosis: Assess a lactate level and prepare to give fluid

   b. Metabolic alkalosis: Assess the pain level and administer analgesics

   c. Respiratory acidosis: Place on lung protective ventilation to prevent lung injury

   d. Respiratory alkalosis: Assess breath sounds and order a stat CXR

14. A 62-year-old patient admitted with Prinzmetal's angina will like be treated with which class of drug relieve coronary vasospasm?

    a. ACE Inhibitor

    b. Beta blocker

    c. Calcium Channel blocker

    d. Vasopressor

15. Your patient with cardiogenic shock is ventilated on 70% FiO_2 and has a Hgb of 7.8 g/dL. Which of the following parameters evaluates tissue oxygenation?

    a. PAOP 14 mm Hg

    b. Cardiac output 3.6 L/min

    c. SvO_2 38%

    d. SVR 1848 dynes/sec/cm^{-5}

16. A 78-year-old female presents to the ED with substernal chest pain and dyspnea. The patient has no history of heart disease. The day prior to her symptom development, she received tragic news that her son and granddaughter were killed in a car accident.

    A 12 lead ECG was performed and revealed deep T wave inversion with a prolonged QT interval. On admission to the ICU, the Troponin level was .06 mcg/L. The echocardiogram revealed left ventricular apical ballooning, dyskinesia, systolic dysfunction, and an ejection fraction of 20%. Coronary angiogram revealed clear coronary arteries. Which type of heart failure do you suspect the patient was experiencing?

    a. Hypertrophic Cardiomyopathy

    b. Takotsubo Cardiomyopathy

    c. Restrictive Cardiomyopathy

    d. Diastolic Heart Failure

17. While caring for a patient with new onset atrial fibrillation who is receiving IV heparin, you notice a steady decline in his platelet count. The patient's initial platelet count was 80,000/mcL. Four days later the platelet count dropped to 35,000/mcL. A lower extremity venous duplex reveals a deep vein thrombosis. The nurse should suspect which of the following?

   a. Pulmonary embolism

   b. Antiphospholipid antibody syndrome

   c. Low platelets are an expected finding when receiving IV heparin

   d. Heparin induced thrombocytopenia (HIT)

18. A patient presents with a STEMI to a hospital that does not have a cardiac catheterization lab & is not able to be transferred to a PCI capable hospital in a timely manner. The decision is made to administer fibrinolytic therapy. What is the appropriate duration for frequent neurological assessment after receiving thrombolytics?

   a. 6 hours

   b. 12 hours

   c. 24 hours

   d. 48 hours

19. A 58 year old female with coronary artery disease and end stage renal disease is admitted to the ICU s/p emergent bowel resection. She uses peritoneal dialysis to manage ESRD at home. She is hemodynamically stable with a 5 liter fluid excess. Crackles are auscultated through her mid lung fields. The serum potassium is 5.6. How should the fluid overload be managed while in the hospital?

a. Provide peritoneal dialysis keeping her same home regimen

b. Begin continuous renal replacement therapy (CRRT)

c. Intermittent hemodialysis

d. No treatment required during this acute phase

20. Which leads are the best for general bedside ECG monitoring in patients with acute coronary syndrome involving the inferior wall of the left ventricle?

a. V1 and II

b. V1 and aVF

c. V3 and I

d. V1 and III

Quiz 4 – Answers

1. A. Decrease the sensitivity (mV) value. In demand mode such as VVI, if the pacemaker fires during the refractory period immediately following the QRS, the pacemaker is under-sensing. This means it cannot "see" or sense the intrinsic rhythm. There are pacing spikes where they shouldn't be—the sensitivity is set toward "least sensitive".

To increase the pacemaker sensitivity (so it sees/senses the QRS), decrease the mV setting. The sensitivity setting (mV) is too high (toward least sensitive or asynchronous mode). Decrease sensitivity setting/number (mV), making the pacemaker more sensitive! Sensitivity settings generally range from 0.5 mV (most sensitive) to 20 mV (least sensitive).

2. D. Balloon inflation occurs at the dicrotic notch and deflation at end diastole. To ensure proper timing, systolic pressure following balloon deflation is lower as a result of afterload reduction. Timing balloon inflation prior to the dicrotic notch can reduce stroke volume with early closure of the aortic valve.

Deflation timing should be done to achieve the lowest possible pressure, about 5 - 10 mm Hg below the unassisted diastole. Late deflation can cause an increased afterload due to the balloon still being inflate while the ventricle is trying to eject blood. We call this "stepping on systole"!

3. A. Troponin-I of 1.5 mcg/L. Differential diagnosis between unstable angina and NSTEMI (NSTE-ACS) includes positive cardiac markers (Troponin-I specifically) to confirm presence of NSTEMI. Cardiac biomarkers can be elevated related to multiple diagnosis.

ST elevation in aVR may be seen with NSTEMI and can be indicative of left main artery stenosis when multiple leads have ST segment depression. NSAIDS are only recommended for pericarditis (inflammatory) pain.

4. C. "As long as I am exercising, having a few drinks every day is ok." This statement requires further clarification and intervention by the nurse. Diet, exercise, and weight management are primary interventions to manage and reduce blood pressure. Alcohol consumption should be limited and consumed in strict moderation.

5. B. Apply defibrillation pads and turn on the defibrillator. CPR is in progress and should not be interrupted. The nurse's priority is to apply the defibrillation pads & defibrillator to assess for a shockable rhythm. Assisted ventilations are important, though defibrillation is a priority. Epinephrine is not a first line therapy in a pulseless patient. Chest compressions and defibrillation (if in a shockable rhythm) are a higher priority.

6. C. Inferior wall MI. An inferior wall MI will present with ST elevation in II, II, aVF & reciprocal changes in I & aVL. Concerns for nausea, vomiting, and risks for heart rhythm changes including bradycardia, second degree AV block Type I (Wenckebach) and RV failure.

Dysrhythmias are a relatively common complication of inferior wall MIs. Both ventricles are innervated by the vagus nerve. When these areas become injured, there is often strong parasympathetic stimulation which can lead to sinus bradycardia or high-grade AV blocks (Wenckebach).

7. D. Doppler ultrasound. Doppler ultrasound is the standard for diagnosis of a DVT. There should be high suspicion for a deep vein thrombosis (DVT). A lower extremity ultrasound will be appropriate to confirm the presence or absence of a DVT. The D-Dimer is sensitive for blood clotting, but not specific to DVT.

The CBC will not reveal specific signs of a clotting disorder. A chest x-ray is not indicated because the chief complaint is the patient's leg.

8. A. Send a complete blood count (CBC). Heparin induced thrombocytopenia should be suspected. HIT is an immune mediated adverse drug reaction caused by antibodies that develop with exposure to Heparin. Petechiae development is a clinical manifestation of heparin induced thrombocytopenia.

Platelets become activated leading to a major risk of thrombosis formation. Sending a CBC with a focus on the platelet count is a priority for diagnosis. HIT should always be suspected with a platelet count that has dropped by 50% after exposure to heparin.

9. A. Discontinuation of the pulmonary artery catheter. A ruptured balloon is suspected. The pulmonary artery catheter needs to be removed.

10. C. Ensure the balloon is deflated and pull back until a PA waveform is observed. During the patient repositioning, the PA catheter has been advanced to the pulmonary capillary bed and is in a permanent "wedge" or occlusive position. As an immediate safety measure the catheter should be pulled back through the sterile sleeve to the pulmonary artery, as this may cause a pulmonary ischemia or a small pulmonary infarction. The PA catheter position will need to be verified by the provider.

11. C. Prepare to transcutaneous pace. Transcutaneous pacing is the initial treatment in a patient who is symptomatic with Complete Heart Block (CHB). Fluids may temporarily increase the BP, but will not change the underlying conduction abnormality of CHB. The patient may not tolerate fluids and can go into heart failure. Atropine is not the drug of choice as it works solely on the SA node. Because there is no communication between the atrium and the ventricle, speeding up the SA node will not improve ventricular conduction. Epinephrine may increase the ventricular rate short term or may also cause arrhythmias.

12. B. Spironolactone. Spironolactone is an aldosterone antagonist, also known as a "K^+ sparing diuretic" and should be used with caution in combination with an ACE inhibitor. Inhibitors of the renin-angiotensin-aldosterone system (RAAS) and mineralocorticoid receptor antagonist (MCRA), they both require close electrolyte monitoring because when combined, put patients at higher risk for hyperkalemia.

13. C. Respiratory acidosis: Place on lung protective ventilation to prevent lung injury. This ABG is indicative of respiratory acidosis with a low pH and elevated $PaCO_2$. In addition, the PaO_2 is low with a P/F ratio of 85. Coupled with the pulmonary contusion, she is at a high risk for developing ARDS. This patient needs to be supported with lung protective ventilation (LPV). LPV utilizes lower tidal volume, starting at 6 mL/kg of predicted body weight (PBW) and PEEP to improve oxygenation.

14. C. Calcium Channel Blocker. Prinzmetal's angina is caused by coronary artery vasospasm. Calcium Channel Blockers such as Amlodipine, Nifedipine, Verapamil & Diltiazem relax smooth muscle in blood vessels and cause coronary vasodilation. They are often combined with nitrates such as isosorbide dinitrate or isosorbide mononitrate to hopefully relieve coronary vasospasm.

15. C. SvO_2 38%. SvO_2 is considered a mixed venous measure and indicates how oxygen is delivered and consumed from the tissues. The goal SvO_2 is 65% - 80% in most patients.

The PAOP is an indirect measurement of the filling pressure (preload) of the left atrium. Cardiac output (C.O.) is a measure of the contractility of the heart, while the systemic vascular resistance (SVR) is a measure of resistance the heart must overcome to eject.

16. B. Takotsubo Cardiomyopathy. Takotsubo (stress induced) Cardiomyopathy is characterized by transient systolic dysfunction of the apical segment of the left ventricle (LV), LV apical ballooning, electrocardiographic changes, mild elevation of Troponin, and absence of obstructive coronary artery disease.

17. D. Heparin induced thrombocytopenia (HIT). The 4 T's score is routinely used to estimate a patient's likelihood of HIT. The 4 T's Score can help identify the patient's risk and if necessary stopping all heparin related therapies. The 4 T's Score includes: thrombocytopenia, timing of the platelet count fall, thrombosis or other new clinical finding possibly associated with heparin and other causes for thrombocytopenia.

In patients who have a confirmed diagnosis of HIT, venous thrombosis is present approximately 20% – 50% of the time. A HIT antibody panel should be done, but is time consuming and typically takes > 24 hours to obtain results.

18. C. 24 hours. Patients treated with fibrinolytic therapy are at risk for bleeding complications including intracranial hemorrhage. Most intracranial hemorrhages occur within the first 24 hours after treatment. Neurologic assessment should be performed regularly for the first 24 hours.

19. C. Intermittent hemodialysis. Because the patient had emergent abdominal surgery, peritoneal dialysis is not an option until she fully heals. CRRT is not indicated as the patient is hemodynamically stable. She needs therapy for the 3 liter volume excess and to treat electrolyte disturbances. A temporary catheter should be placed and the patient treated with intermittent hemodialysis.

20. D. V1 and III. The V lead can be moved across the precordium to monitor dysrhythmias (V1) or placed over the injured myocardial wall. Ischemia is detected by ST changes. Lead III provides the most direct view of the inferior wall which is supplied by the RCA. Lead III is a far more sensitive monitoring lead than the traditional lead II view.

Quiz 5 – Questions

1. The nurse is caring for a pacemaker dependent patient with a newly placed transvenous pacemaker. The bedside ECG tracing reveals pacer spikes without subsequent ventricular contraction. Which action should the nurse prioritize?

    a. Increase the mA

    b. Change the battery

    c. Order a STAT chest radiograph

    d. Obtain serum electrolytes and cardiac markers

2. In the development of a plan of care for a patient with a new IABP, the nurse includes which of the following to ensure effectiveness of balloon pump timing?

    a. Proper position of the head of the bed above 45 degrees

    b. Frequent assessment for changes in serum electrolytes

    c. Reevaluate timing only after a change in heart rate by 50 beats per minute

    d. Verifying the absence of a trigger signal for the IABP console

3. A patient presents to the Emergency Department with sudden, sharp, stabbing substernal chest pain that is improved by sitting up & leaning forward. A pericardial friction rub is auscultated. A 12 lead ECG is performed and reveals concave ST segment elevation with PR segment depression in all leads. Cardiac biomarkers are within normal limits. Which of the following is suspected?

    a. Pleural effusion

    b. Pulmonary embolism

    c. Myocardial ischemia

    d. Pericarditis

4. The nurse is preparing a patient for discharge after admission for a STEMI with PCI and stent placement to the left anterior descending (LAD) artery. Which discharge order should the nurse question?

   a. Discontinue aspirin & begin Plavix 100 mg daily
   b. Metoprolol (Lopressor) 12.5 mg BID
   c. Simvastatin 20 mg at bedtime
   d. Lisinopril 5 mg every am

5. An 18-year-old patient is receiving Targeted Temperature Management (TTM) after resuscitation from a cardiac arrest. His current temperature is 33.4°C. The presence of bigeminal PVCs are noted on the bedside monitor. Which action is a priority?

   a. Assess serum electrolytes
   b. Change the ECG electrodes
   c. Administer medication to minimize shivering
   d. Perform a neurologic exam

6. The Rapid Response Team arrives to the Telemetry Unit to assess a patient complaining of chest and back pain rated as "8 out of 10". Patient vital signs are as follows:

   HR 60
   BP 88/42 (57)
   RR 16

   A 12 Lead ECG shows ST segment depression with tall R waves in V1 & V2 and no other changes visible. What is the appropriate next action to take?

a. Place ECG leads below the left scapula & obtain a Posterior ECG
   b. Send serum cardiac biomarkers
   c. Administer 325 mg Aspirin chewable to the patient
   d. Have the patient cough and lean forward

7. Your patient is being consented for a MAZE procedure to treat atrial fibrillation. Which statement by the patient demonstrates a correct understanding of the procedure?
   a. "My heart function will be weaker."
   b. "I will never have an irregular heart beat again."
   c. "The scar tissue that develops will change how irregular beats travel though my heart."
   d. "My heart muscle will be shocked to limit irregular beats."

8. The nurse is discontinuing a femoral artery procedural sheath with a preceptor for the first time. Which statement by the nurse requires additional education by the preceptor?
   a. "The goal ACT prior to removal is < 150 seconds."
   b. "Frequent assessments of circulation in the extremity after removal are a nursing priority."
   c. "If we remove the sheath with an ACT > 150 seconds, we will just have to hold pressure longer."
   d. "Hematomas can develop in the groin site from where the sheath was pulled."

9. A patient in the ICU with Cardiomyopathy has sudden onset weakness in the right upper and lower extremities and slurred speech. Vital signs are as follows:

   HR 92

   BP 90/42 (58)

   RR 28

   SpO_2 92% on 2 L NC

   An emergent CT scan of the head reveals the absence of an intracranial hemorrhage. Which order should the nurse anticipate next?

   a. Heparin infusion

   b. Coumadin 5 mg PO

   c. Alteplase (Activase) IV infusion

   d. Hourly neurologic assessments

10. Your patient is admitted to the Cardiac Intensive Care Unit with progressive dyspnea and systolic heart failure. A right heart catheterization reveals a cardiac index of 1.6 L/min/m². Which of the following home medications should be held on admission?

    a. Digitalis (digoxin)

    b. Spironolactone

    c. Bumetanide (bumex)

    d. Carvedilol (Coreg)

11. You are caring for a 54-year-old female after repair of a femur fracture. She has a history of atrial fibrillation, DVTs and anxiety. She has leg pain and is having difficulty breathing. You notice her O_2 saturation is 90% and is breathing 36 bpm. She is in atrial fibrillation at a rate of 132/minute and her BP is 94/60 (71). You medicate her for pain with no change in her vital signs, RR or O_2 sat.

Next, you notify the provider because you are concerned for which of the following reasons?

a. She has inadequate pain relief

b. She missed her morning dose Amiodarone, explaining the tachycardia

c. She may need her home dose of Ativan for anxiety

d. She is at high risk of Pulmonary Embolism

12. You are caring for a patient with substernal chest pain. You assess a 12 lead ECG and notice ST segment elevation in leads II, III & aVF. Next, a right-sided ECG is obtained revealing ST segment elevation in leads V4R, V5R, V6R.

Vital signs:

HR 106

BP 86/42

RR 18

SpO_2 96%

Which of the following interventions should be initiated?

a. Lactated Ringers 500 ml IV bolus

b. Metoprolol 5 mg IV push x 3

c. Lasix 40 mg IV

d. Sublingual Nitroglycerin, followed by an IV infusion

13. A 54-year-old was admitted after recent dental work with fever, dyspnea and pleuritic pain. He has been diagnosed with Infective Endocarditis (IE) of his prosthetic mitral valve.

Where would you expect to hear a murmur when auscultating his heart sounds?

    a. The fourth and fifth intercostal spaces along the left sternal edge

    b. The second intercostal space along the left sternal border

    c. Fifth intercostal space at the left midclavicular line (cardiac apex)

    d. The right sternal border second intercostal space

14. You are caring for 54-year-old male admitted with Sepsis. The initial resuscitation has been administered.

Vital signs are as follows:

HR 110 in Sinus Tachycardia

BP 84/52 (62)

T 100°F

RR 20

He has an arterial line & is mechanically ventilated on Assist Control mode, Vt 8 ml/kg, Rate 20, 60% F_iO_2, PEEP +10. Which of the following parameters indicate the patient may be responsive to additional fluid?

    a. CVP 12 mm Hg

    b. Arterial pulse pressure variability of 18%

    c. Lactate 2.4 mmol/L

    d. Urine output 40 mL/hour

15. A 53-year-old patient with a history of diabetes, heart failure and CAD presents with lethargy, nausea and fever. The Troponin-I level is 3.6 with ST depression in multiple leads on the 12 Lead ECG. A NSTEMI is diagnosed.

Vital signs:

HR 120

BP 110/60 (76)

RR 42

ABG results:

pH 7.19

$PaCO_2$ 28

PaO_2 65

HCO_3 15

SaO_2 92%

Other labs:

Na^+ 132, K^+ 2.6, Cl^- 92, CO_2 18, Glucose 648

Which of the following treatments should be prioritized?

a. IV fluids & IV potassium replacement

b. IV insulin infusion & IV fluids

c. Sodium bicarbonate & potassium infusion

d. Diuretic & insulin infusion

16. Your patient is complaining of stabbing substernal chest pain that she rates as "10 out of 10". The monitor shows a narrow complex rhythm at a rate of 125 beats per minute. The blood pressure is 82/40 (57) mm Hg. The pulse oximetry reads 95% on room air. The 12 Lead ECG reveals ST elevation in leads II, III, aVF & V1. Which of the following medications should be used to treat her hypotension?

a. Lisinopril

b. Morphine

c. Nitroglycerin

d. 1 Liter of IV fluid

17. Which of the following patient characteristics meet criteria for cardiac resynchronization therapy (CRT) for a patient with left ventricular systolic dysfunction?

    a. EF 52%, QRS 150 ms, NYHA functional class II

    b. EF 44%, QRS 130 ms, NYHA functional class II

    c. EF 29%, QRS 155 ms, NYHA functional class II

    d. EF 45%, RBBB, and NYHA class III

18. A 65-year-old female presents to the Emergency Department with progressively worsening orthopnea, paroxysmal nocturnal dyspnea, chest pain, and early satiety. She reports her brother passed away suddenly about two weeks ago. She has no history of cardiovascular disease.

    A 12 Lead ECG is performed and shows ST elevation in leads V_1 - V_3 and a prolonged QT interval. The Troponin-I level is mildly elevated. Left heart catheterization does not show obstructive disease. Left ventriculography demonstrates apical ballooning and hypercontraction of the basal segments.

    These findings are most consistent with:

    a. Acute pericarditis

    b. Coronary artery vasospasm

    c. Hypertrophic Cardiomyopathy

    d. Takotsubo Cardiomyopathy

19. You admit a 33-year-old male to the ICU from the Emergency Department with Status Asthmaticus. He is receiving supplemental oxygen via face mask and has received continuous nebulized bronchodilators & anticholinergics. Which of the following medications is indicated for this patient?

a. IV beta blockers

b. Antibiotics

c. Steroids

d. Anxiolytics

20. You are caring for a 56 year old woman admitted with thyrotoxicosis. Which of the following dysrhythmias commonly occurs with hyperthyroidism?

a. Atrial fibrillation

b. Torsade de Pointes

c. 2nd degree type 2 heart block

d. Ventricular tachycardia

Quiz 5 – Answers

1. A. Increase the mA. Loss of capture for a pacemaker dependent patient is a medical emergency. Contributing factors for loss of capture include changes in myocardial tissue oxygenation & electrolyte abnormalities, fibrin clot on the catheter tip, or malposition of the catheter. Acidosis can also affect capture of the pacing stimulus. However, the priority is to ensure capture and proper conduction by increasing the energy or the mA.

2. B. Frequent assessment for changes in serum electrolytes. The risk of cardiac rhythm irregularities can significantly impact IABP timing. Frequent assessment of electrolytes are within can decrease the chance of rhythm irregularities. Proper head of the bed position to up to 30 degrees. Timing should be reevaluated after heart rate changes of 10 - 20 beats per minute and the trigger signal always verified. Electrodes may be changed to ensure a proper signal.

3. D. Pericarditis. Pericarditis is an inflammation of the pericardium. It can be caused by an inflammatory response after a myocardial infarction or by a viral or bacterial infection. Clinical signs include chest pain that is aggravated with position changes or deep breathing. Often a friction rub will be heard on auscultation. ST segment elevation occurs because of the involvement in the underlying epicardium. ST depression may be localized in V_1 and aVR.

A few considerations to differentiate between pericarditis and a STEMI; PR depression is generally transient in pericarditis and most commonly seen in viral pericarditis.

4. A. Discontinue aspirin & begin Plavix 100 mg daily. This should be questioned by the nurse. Standard discharge medications post MI include ASA and P2Y12 inhibitor therapy in combination. ACE inhibitors, beta blockers and statins are all indicated in the current guidelines.

5. A. Assess serum electrolytes. During TTM, electrolytes shift significantly and can have an effect on cardiac rhythm & function. This is especially true during the induction & maintenance phases of cooling. It is important to ensure potassium, magnesium, & calcium are at therapeutic levels. During cooling therapy potassium and magnesium are often deficient due to cellular shifting & should be replaced. As the patient is rewarmed, electrolyte replacement should be discontinued as electrolytes will shift back into the serum.

6. A. Place ECG leads below the left scapula & obtain a Posterior ECG. With ST depression & tall R waves in leads V1 & V2, this may represent a reciprocal change for a posterior wall MI. The appropriate next step is to obtain a Posterior ECG to evaluate for ST segment elevation in V7 - V9. Place the three ECG leads subscapular on the left back, moving medial with lead placement.

7. C. "The scar tissue that develops will change how irregular beats travel through my heart." In a MAZE procedure, a series of incisions are made to the right and left atria in a maze pattern. The idea is as scar tissue develops, the electrical conduction & circuits would be blocked by the scar tissue alleviating atrial fibrillation.

8. C. "If we remove the sheath with an ACT > 150 seconds, we will just have to hold pressure longer." To ensure the patient safety, sheaths are not removed until the activated clotting time (ACT) is < 150 seconds. ACTs are maintained between 300 - 350 seconds safely for therapeutic management of anticoagulation. All of the other statements indicate the nurse understand concepts regarding sheath removal.

9. C. Alteplase (Activase) IV infusion. Alteplase (rtPA) is the only approved antithrombotic for stroke and should be administered within one hour of the identification of stroke symptoms. This is known as "door to needle" time.

A complete National Institute of Health (NIH) neurologic assessment will need to be completed before & after administration of Alteplase. Generally neurologic assessments will be more frequent than hourly due to the risk of hemorrhagic conversion of an ischemic stroke. Contraindications to Alteplase include recent major surgery, severe HTN, stroke, ICH and head trauma.

10. D. Carvedilol (Coreg). Carvedilol (Coreg), metoprolol (Lopressor) & Bisoprolol (Zebeta) are three common beta blockers used for goal directed medical management for both systolic and diastolic heart failure. During an episode of acute decompensated heart failure (due to volume overload or worsening global cardiac function), the patient may require a positive inotrope infusion, like Dobutamine or Milrinone.

Beta blockers have negative inotropic effects that decrease contractility. In this exacerbated condition, the patient requires augmented contractility to treat the low cardiac output. Holding the beta blocker is beneficial to increase contractility and treat acute decompensated heart failure. After aggressive diuresis and "tuning up", the Carvedilol should be restarted.

11. D. She is at high risk of Pulmonary Embolism. The patient has a history of atrial fibrillation and DVTs and is at a high risk for Pulmonary Embolism (PE). While pain and anxiety could be contributing factors and should be addressed, the risk for PE should be the primary concern given her low O_2 sat and increased RR. Pain and anxiety are likely signs of DVT & PE.

12. A. Lactated Ringers 500 ml IV bolus. This patient is exhibiting signs of a right ventricular MI. Beta blockers can reduce heart rate and contractility slowing AV conduction and significantly reduce preload. Because patients with a right ventricular MI are preload dependent, nitrates, morphine & diuretics should all be avoided. IV fluid is the most appropriate initial intervention and should be administered to increase preload and forward flow to the left side of the heart.

13. C. Fifth intercostal space at the left midclavicular line (cardiac apex). The mitral valve is best auscultated over the 5th intercostal space in the mid clavicular line at the cardiac apex. The other answers are the best for the following valves: a. tricuspid, b. pulmonic & d. aortic.

14. B. Arterial pulse pressure variability of 18%. Pulse pressure variability is a marker of the variation in cardiac output during inspiration and expiration. If cardiac output varies more with respiration, the patient is likely to respond to fluid.

Normal pulse pressure variability is 10 - 13%. As a patient on positive pressure ventilation inhales, intrathoracic pressure increases. This increase can compress the inferior vena cava, decreasing venous blood return. On an arterial line this is seen are a variation in the wave itself. If the variability is > 13%, the patient will likely be fluid responsive. If the variability is < 10%, a vasopressor should be used to treat hypotension.

15. A. IV fluids & IV potassium replacement. This patient is in Diabetic Ketoacidosis (DKA) and hydration is the priority intervention followed by correction of hyperglycemia and electrolytes. The potassium is critically low and must be replaced before insulin is initiated. In general, the K^+ should be above 3.5 before an insulin infusion is started. Insulin will push potassium into the cell worsening the serum potassium concentration. This could potentially lead to life threatening dysrhythmias.

16. D. 1 Liter of IV fluid. When tachycardia is present in the setting of an inferior MI, a right-sided ECG should be performed to rule out RV infarction. RV infarction or ischemia may occur in up to 50% of patients with an inferior wall MI. Patients with RV dysfunction and acute infarction are dependent on maintenance of RV "filling" pressure or preload to maintain cardiac output. Thus, nitrates, diuretics, and other vasodilators (ACE inhibitors) should be avoided because severe hypotension may result. Hypotension is initially treated with an IV fluid bolus.

17. C. EF 29%, QRS 155 ms, NYHA functional class II. Patients with a left ventricular ejection fraction (EF) < 35% and a QRS duration > 150 ms with a LBBB have been shown to receive the most benefit from CRT. Patients with a QRS duration of 130 – 150 ms and a non-LBBB pattern are also considered if they are failing goal directed medical therapy for heart failure.

18. D. Takotsubo Cardiomyopathy. Takotsubo Cardiomyopathy is also known as "Stress Induced Cardiomyopathy", "Broken Heart Syndrome" or "Apical Ballooning Syndrome." Takotsubo Cardiomyopathy has the highest incidence in postmenopausal women. The exact mechanism is not fully understood. There is a strong correlation with physical or emotional distress, thus postulating a catecholamine induced vasospasm causing myocardial stunning. Standard heart failure medications are used to treat Takotsubo. Coronary vasospasm may be the cause of the regional wall motion abnormality, but the compilation of clinical data given is more accurately described as Takotsubo Cardiomyopathy. Most patients recover within a few months.

19. C. Steroids. In addition to $Beta_2$ agonism like albuterol, steroids are very important in the management of Status Asthmaticus. Steroids decrease inflammation which leads to decreased mucus production, improved oxygenation and reduction of beta-agonist requirements.

Routine administration of antibiotics is not recommended unless there is evidence of infection. Beta blockers are not indicated and should be avoided in asthmatics if possible. Patients may also benefit from small doses of anxiolytics; however, they should be used judiciously.

20. Atrial fibrillation. Between 10% - 15% of patients with hyperthyroid issues develop atrial fibrillation. This incidence increases with age irrespective of associated heart disease.

References

2020 ACC/AHA Guideline for the Management of Patients With Valvular Heart Disease: A Report of the American College of Cardiology/American Heart Association Joint Committee on Clinical Practice Guidelines. Circulation;143(5)

2020 American Heart Association Guidelines for Cardiopulmonary Resuscitation and Emergency Cardiovascular Care. Circulation. Volume 142, Issue 16_Suppl_2, 20 October 2020; Pages S337-S357 https://doi.org/10.1161/CIR.0000000000000918

2021 AHA/ACC/ASE/CHEST/SAEM/SCCT/SCMR Guideline for the Evaluation and Diagnosis of Chest Pain: A Report of the American College of Cardiology/American Heart Association Joint Committee on Clinical Practice Guidelines. Circulation;144(22)

2021 Guideline for the Prevention of Stroke in Patients With Stroke and Transient Ischemic Attack: A Guideline From the American Heart Association/American Stroke Association. Stroke;52(7)

2022 AHA/ACC/HFSA Guideline for the Management of Heart Failure: A Report of the American College of Cardiology/American Heart Association Joint Committee on Clinical Practice Guidelines. J Am Coll Cardiol 2022

Effects of Early Empagliflozin Initiation on Diuresis and Kidney Function in Patients With Acute Decompensated Heart Failure (EMPAG-HF). Circulation 2022;Jun 29

Aehlert, Barbara. *ECGs Made Easy*, 6th edition. Elsevier; 2018.

Burns, S.M. & Delgado, S.A. (2018). *AACN Essentials of Critical Care Nursing*, 4th edition. McGraw-Hill Education.

Cardiothoracic Critical Care – Sidebotham, McKee, Gillham, Levy

Coutre S, MD. Clinical presentation and diagnosis of heparin-induced thrombocytopenia. UpToDate. Waltham, MA: UpToDate Inc. http://uptodate.com (accessed January 8, 2018).

Gahart BL, Nazareno AR. 2015 *Intravenous medications*. 31st ed. St. Louis, MO: Mosby/Elsevier; 2015.

Hardin, S.R., & Kaplow, R. (2018). *Cardiac Surgery: Essentials for Critical Care Nursing*. (3rd ed.). Jones & Bartlett Learning

Jacobson, C. Marzlin, K., Webner, C. 2021. *Cardiovascular Nursing Practice: Cardiovascular Essentials*, 3rd Edition.

Jacobson, C, Marzlin, K & Webner, C. 2021. *Cardiovascular Nursing Practice: Cardiac Arrhythmias and 12 Lead ECG Interpretation*, 3rd edition.

Lough ME. Hemodynamic Monitoring: Evolving Technologies and Clinical Practice. St. Louis, MO: Mosby/Elsevier; 2016.

Outcomes after Angiography with Sodium Bicarbonate and Acetylcysteine. *New England Journal of Medicine* 2017, November 12. PMID: 29130810.

Perpetua, E. & Keegan, P. (2021). 7th edition *Cardiac Nursing.* Wolters Kluwer/Lippincott, Williams, & Wilkins: Philadelphia, PA

Sole ML, Klein DG, Moseley MJ. *Introduction to Critical Care Nursing.* 8th ed. Philadelphia, PA: Saunders/ Elsevier; 2021.

Wiegand, D.L-M. (2017). *AACN: Procedure Manual for Critical Care.* (7th ed.). Saunders/Elsevier: St. Louis, MO.

Urden L, Stacy KM, Lough ME. *Priorities in Critical Care Nursing.* 8th ed. St. Louis, MO: Mosby/Elsevier; 2021.

About the author...

Nicole Kupchik has practiced as a Critical Care nurse for over twenty-five years. She obtained a Nursing Degree from Purdue University in 1993 and a Master of Nursing from the University of Washington in 2008.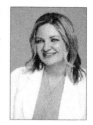

Nicole's nursing career began in the Chicago area. From 1995 to 1998, she journeyed across the United States as a traveling nurse, after which she landed in Seattle. Her first job in Seattle was in the Cardiothoracic Intensive Care Unit (5 SE) at the University of Washington. In 2001, she began working at Harborview Medical Center—a change that spurred an interest in resuscitation.

Shortly thereafter, Nicole was part of a multidisciplinary team that was one of the first in the United States to implement therapeutic hypothermia after cardiac arrest. As part of this effort, Nicole was responsible for protocol development and has published numerous papers on this topic.

In 2008, Nicole was part of a team that implemented a formalized Sepsis program at Harborview. The program resulted in a reduction in mortality, hospital length of stay and significant cost avoidance. She collaborated with IT specialists to develop innovative methods to electronically screen hospitalized patients in acute care units for sepsis. For this work, the program was awarded two Patient Safety & Clinical Leadership awards.

In 2002, Nicole obtained certification as a CCRN®. She admittedly attended three certification review courses before finally taking the exam! Once she passed the exam she questioned why she hesitated and lacked confidence to sit the exam. Shortly thereafter, Nicole began teaching segments of CCRN® certification review courses at her hospital. In 2006, she started co-teaching courses nationally.

In 2013, Nicole founded Nicole Kupchik Consulting & Education. She frequently teaches review courses nationally. She holds certification as a CCNS®, CCRN®, PCCN® & CMC®.

Her courses are well attended and often sell out! Her wit and sense of humor make the course interesting & entertaining. Nicole has a gift of being able to break information down in a way that is really easy to understand. She hopes to instill confidence in nurses that they can do it!

OTHER BOOKS BY NICOLE KUPCHIK

Critical Care Survival Guide
Ace the CCRN®: You Can Do It! Study Guide
Ace the CCRN®: You Can Do It! Practice Review Questions
Ace the PCCN®: You Can Do It! Study Guide
Ace the PCCN®: You Can Do It! Practice Review Questions
Ace the CSC®: You Can Do It! Study Guide with Practice Review Questions

Nicole also has online courses available for
the CCRN®, PCCN®, CMC® & CSC® exams!

FOLLOW NICOLE ON SOCIAL MEDIA:

👍 Nicole Kupchik Consulting & Education

📷 @nicolekupchik

♪ @nicolekupchik

▶ YouTube Nicole Kupchik

You Can Do It!

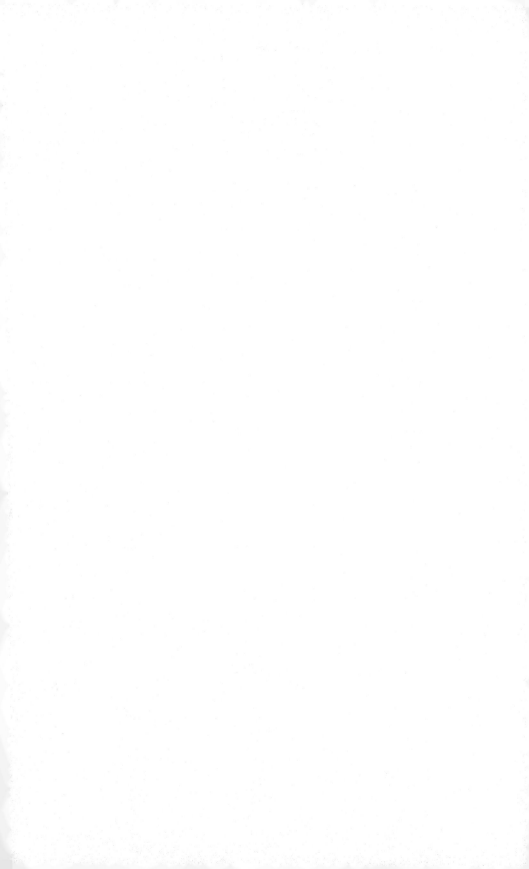

Made in the USA
Las Vegas, NV
12 July 2024

92169952R00144